Table

Dedicated to healthcare professionals worldwide.

Correspondence:

Behind the Knife: The Surgery Podcast
btkpodcast@gmail.com
www.behindtheknife.org
Twitter: @BehindTheKnife

Authors:

Kevin Kniery, MD, MPH

Jason Bingham, MD

John McClellan, MD

Scott Steele, MD, MBA

Meghana Kashyap, MD

Michael Vu, MD

Illustrations:

Irene Yu, MD

Acknowledgements:

Matthew J. Martin, MD

Woo Do, MD

Shreya Gupta, MD

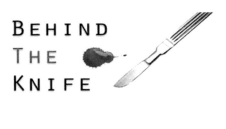

BEHIND
THE
KNIFE

Preface

- These outlines are the culmination of notes we have compiled over the years in our own preparation for the ABSITE. They are also the basis for the BTK podcast ABSITE review series. As such, they are intended to serve as a companion study aid to the podcast series.

- We have done our best to ensure the accuracy of the information within the outlines as well as the podcast. However, we cannot guarantee you will pass your boards solely with the information provided here, nor is this review intended for direct clinical use or a substitute for clinical competency.

Why BTK Board Review?

- We know how to study for this test, and we know what it takes to do well. We are sharing with you our notes from over the years.

- Our review is approachable, concise, and convenient. It is clinically based and more up to date with current guidelines when compared to other reviews on the market.

- It is effective to learn via different formats and repetition is key. This review rounds out what's already available and augments what we discuss in the audio review.

What This Review Is:

- A thorough review of current clinical management guidelines for the most commonly tested surgical topics.

- Designed to be reviewed multiple times in order to:
  o Help you score well on the ABSITE.

- Help you pass the general surgery Qualifying Exam and Certifying Exam.
- Help you prepare for clerkships, rotations, and daily rounds.

What This Review Isn't:

- This is not surgical trivia – Most currently available study guides are heavy in basic science minutia. We are not going to tell you the components of the coagulation cascade. We are going to focus on key components of clinical management of surgical disease based on current guideline. This is the direction the general surgery boards are going, and there is less and less basic science showing up on the ABSITE and the boards.
  - Other review books will tell you that the APC gene is on chromosome 5, but will they tell you what the current guidelines say regarding the surgical management of the axilla with node positive breast CA? Probably not, but we will.

- This is not an exhaustive study guide. This is simply what we view as the most distilled down, high yield, need to know information for the ABSITE and the general surgery boards.

How We Recommend You Prepare For The Boards:

- Study year round – Strive to be excellent at your job – Dominate each day. There is no replacement for this. You can't slack all year and expect to dominate the ABSITE/Boards.

- That being said – it's a test and there is gamesmanship to doing well on it. Many excellent residents and surgeons struggle with the boards. So, being smart and good at your job isn't enough. This is where our review can help.

- Start dedicated ABSITE/Board studying at least 4-6 weeks prior to the test. Things you'll need:
  - A Q bank (Several options available) – Do at least 1000 Q's (minimum) – Take notes as you go through questions – Review your notes and then re-do the questions you got wrong
  - BTK ABSITE review – Listen and Re-listen – Listen actively

(try to anticipate the answer before we tell you)

- ○ BTK written review – Use it as a companion to the podcast to reinforce your knowledge.

- Get rest the night before, take snacks, relax, and …
DOMINATE THE DAY!!!

We hope you enjoy this new edition with illustrations, tables, and finally a print option!

01 HEAD AND NECK

High Yield Anatomy

- Name the structures of the thoracic outlet from anterior to posterior
  - ○ Anterior to posterior – Subclavian Vein → Phrenic Nerve → Anterior Scalene → Subclavian Artery (SCA) → Middle Scalene

> The phrenic nerve travels from lateral to medial on top of the anterior scalene as it courses into the chest.

- Name the boundaries and contents of the anterior and posterior neck triangles
  - ○ Anterior neck triangle
    - Anterior boundary— Midline of the neck
    - Posterior boundary — Sternocleidomastoid (SCM)
    - Inferior (Apex) — Sternal notch
    - Superior (Base) — Lower border of the body of the mandible
    - Contents: Carotid Sheath
  - ○ Posterior Neck Triangle
    - Anterior boundary — Posterior border of SCM
    - Posterior boundary — Trapezius muscle
    - Base — Middle 3rd of Clavicle
    - Apex — Intersection of SCM and Trapezius
    - Contents: Spinal Accessory Nerve
  - ○ Anterior/Posterior triangles are broken up into smaller triangles, but these are not commonly tested

- What muscles does the recurrent laryngeal nerve (RLN) innervate? How does the anatomy differ on the right side versus the left side?
  - ○ RLN branches off vagus nerve and innervates muscles of larynx (except for cricothyroid muscle, which is innervated by Superior Laryngeal Nerve)

- Right side: Vagus passes anterior to SCA and the RLN loops behind SCA and travels superiorly in Tracheoesophageal (TE) groove
- Left side: Vagus passes anterior to aortic arch between Left Common Carotid Artery and SCA and RLN then loops behind aortic arch and travels superiorly in TE groove

> The superior laryngeal nerve innervates the cricothyroid muscle, all other laryngeal muscles are innervated by the recurrent laryngeal nerve

Head and Neck Cancers

- What is the most common head and neck cancer?
  - Squamous cell cancer (SCC)
  - 5th most common Cancer overall; Men affected more than women 5:1
  - Risk Factors: Alcohol and tobacco (Synergistic Effect), HPV
  - Each subsite (e.g. oral cavity, oropharynx, nasopharynx, hypopharynx, larynx, nose, paranasal sinus, and salivary gland) has its own staging system and treatment recommendations. However, IN GENERAL:
    - Stage I and II – Local disease (No regional or distant Mets)
    - Stage III and IV – Either locally aggressive or distant mets
    - Surgery or Radiation acceptable for stage I-II. Surgery vs. radiation will depend on location and morbidity of resection (e.g. WLE for intraoral lesions vs radiation for vocal cord lesions).
    - Multimodality required for Stage III-IV. Usually surgery (WLE + MRND) followed by radiation +/- chemotherapy
    - Oral SCC >4cm (or + nodes/bone invasion) needs resection with MRND followed by postop radiation
- Are large or small salivary gland tumors more likely to be malignant, and what are the subtypes of the most common salivary malignant tumors?
  - Tumors of small salivary glands more likely to be malignant

than larger glands (i.e. sublingual > submandibular > parotid)

- o Malignant Tumors
  - Mucoepidermoid Cancer – Most common
    - Treatment → Resection (total parotidectomy with facial nerve preservation if parotid) with MRND, +/- postop XRT
  - Adenoid Cystic Cancer
    - Slow growing with tendency to locally invade (particularly nerves)
    - Tx: resection (total parotidectomy with facial nerve preservation if parotid) with MRND, +/- postop XRT
      - o Don't need to aggressively resect Adenoid Cystic Cancer if it would result in high morbidity as it is very sensitive to XRT

- What are the principles of management of an unknown primary head and neck cancer tumor (i.e. regional metastasis to node without known primary)?
  1. Thorough head and neck exam – included fiberoptic exam of nasopharynx and larynx
  2. FNA of regional node or excisional biopsy
  3. CT scan Head/Neck/Chest +/- PET
  4. OR for direct laryngoscopy, esophagoscopy, and ipsilateral tonsillectomy, + biopsies directed by previous work-up
  - Most common site of unknown primary is tonsil followed by base of tongue
  - If no primary identified – will still need *ipsilateral* MRND and *bilateral* XRT

- How do you diagnose and treat a melanoma of the head and neck?
  - o Diagnose with full-thickness biopsy (excisional, incisional, or punch) – NO SHAVE BIOPSY!
  - o Staged like melanoma at other sites (See melanoma section)

- o Treatment: Resection with the same margins as other sites if possible (1cm for lesions <1mm in depth and 2cm for those >2mm in depth)

  - Tumor margins can be adjusted if abutting critical structures

  - Branches of facial nerve should be preserved unless clinically involved

  - Confirm negative margins prior to reconstruction

  - Moh's surgery also an option, especially if resection would result in morbidity

- o Lymphadenectomy is required if regional nodes are clinically positive.

- o If clinically node negative → Sentinel Lymph Node (SLN) for >1mm depth

- o How to determine lymph node basin for melanoma of head/ neck → Primary lesions anterior to imaginary line from one tragus to the other will drain anteriorly through the parotid basin

  - For anterior lesions → superficial parotidectomy and selective anterior neck dissection

  - For posterior lesions → Selective posterior neck dissection

- o Adjuvant therapy for melanoma is currently undergoing rapid advancement and recommendations may change in near future

  - Adjuvant interferon alpha has been showed survival benefit in advanced disease, however it has many side effects and poorly tolerated

  - Adjuvant radiation therapy may help with regional control, however has no survival benefit

  - Ongoing trials for targeted therapies (monoclonal antibodies, oncogene inhibitors) are showing a lot of promise

Quick Hits

- Painless mass on roof of the mouth?
  - Torus Palatinus (overgrowth of cortical bone)
  - Treatment? Do Nothing (resect if interfering with denture fit)

- Most common site for oral cavity cancer?
  - Lower lip (related to sun exposure)
  - Will need flap reconstruction if > ½ lip resected

- EBV related H&N Cancer?
  - Nasopharyngeal SCC
  - Treatment? → XRT

- MC malignant salivary gland tumor?
  - Mucoepidermoid carcinoma

- MC benign salivary gland tumor? And what is the treatment?
  - Pleomorphic adenoma
  - Superficial Parotidectomy (Do not enucleate this lesion)

- Gustatory sweating following parotidectomy? What is the cause of this?
  - Frey's syndrome
  - Injury to auriculotemporal nerve that then cross innervates with sympathetic fibers

- Elderly patient with postop fever, pain, and swelling at angle of jaw? What is the organism and what is the treatment?
  - Suppurative parotiditis
  - Staphylococcus
  - Hydration and antibiotics; I&D if abscess is present

- Management of bleeding at tracheostomy site?
  - Small amount → Bronchoscopy to rule out Tracheoinnominate fistula
  - Large amount → Place finger into tracheostomy, hold manual pressure against sternum and go to OR emergently for median sternotomy and resection of innominate artery. Close tracheal side primarily and cover with strap muscle (do NOT put synthetic interposition graft. It will get infected and blow out).

02 THYROID

High Yield Anatomy

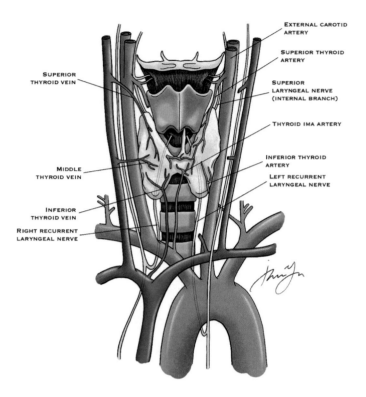

Figure 1: Thyroid Anatomy (Thyroid in Grey)

Vascular supply:
- Superior thyroid artery: branch from External carotid artery

- Inferior thyroid artery: branch off of thyrocervical artery

- Ima artery off of innominate directly to the isthmus

- Superior thyroid vein drains into IJV, inferior drains into innominate vein

Nerves:
- Superior laryngeal nerve: motor to cricothyroid muscle; loss of projection and fatigue

- Recurrent laryngeal nerve: Right travels with vagus and loops around Right innominate artery

- Left travels with vagus and loops around aorta
  - Preoperative laryngoscopy to visualize cords, bilateral damage can obstruct airway

Thyroglobulin: stores T3 (more active) and T4

Thyroid Embryology:
4th Endodermal pouch → Bilobed solid organ---follicular cells, colloid and parafollicular cells (produces calcitonin)
Pyramidal lobe extension can cause thyroglossal duct cyst; resect this as it has the potential to get infected or malignant transformation

High-Yield Pathophysiology/Treatment

- Thyroid storm:
  - Seen in Grave's disease
  - Treatment with beta blockers, Lugol's solution, cooling blankets
- Thyroid Nodule:
  - Ultrasound (Look for hypoechogenecity, microcalcification, irregular margins, unorganized vascular patterns, lymphatic invasion) followed by FNA

• Indeterminant	• Repeat FNA
• Benign	• Repeat US in 6-12 months
• AUS/FLUS	• Repeat FNA
• Follicular neoplasm	• Lobectomy
• Suspicious malignancy	• Lobectomy
• Malignancy	• Total thyroidectomy

Table 1: Bethesda Criteria
*AUS – Atypia of undetermined significance
**FLUS – Follicular lesion of undetermined significance

- Hyperthyroidism:
  - Low TSH, elevated T3, T4
  - Treatment with PTU (side effects of aplastic anemia or agranulocytosis) or methimazole (cretinism, aplastic anemia and agranulocytosis)
  - <u>PTU OK during Pregnancy</u> as it does not cross placenta
- Graves' disease:
  - Diffuse uptake of radioactive iodine (RAI), antibodies against TSH receptors
  - RAI worsens ophthalmopathy
- Multi-nodular goiter:
  - Total or subtotal thyroidectomy
- Thyroiditis:
  - Hashimoto's: caused by <u>antithyroid antibodies</u>; treatment with thyroid replacement
  - Subacute granulomatous: viral etiology, treatment with NSAIDs, steroids
- Papillary thyroid cancer:
  - <u>MC thyroid malignancy</u>; in women; spread lymphatically
  - Biopsy pathology shows psammoma bodies, orphan Annie nucleus
  - Tx with total thyroidectomy with Level VI involvement
    - Do total – so can follow up thyroglobulin for surveillance, postoperative radioiodine treatment, remove potential multifocal disease
- Follicular Thyroid Cancer:
  - FNA is not reliable so do diagnostic/therapeutic lobectomy
  - Hematogenous spread
  - Treatment with total thyroidectomy, MRND for + nodes and postoperative Radioactive iodine ablation

- Medullary Thyroid Cancer:
  - Cancer from parafollicular C cells producing Calcitonin
  - 20% associated with germline mutations in _RET_ oncogene
  - Tx with total thyroidectomy with Central dissection, modified radical dissection if lymph nodes involved
  - Surveillance with CEA, Calcitonin

	Risk	Prophylactic thyroidectomy
MEN2A, MEN2B are associated with medullary thyroid cancer	Low risk (A)	By 5 years of age, may delay if certain criteria are met
	Medium risk (B)	By 5 years of age, may delay if certain criteria are met
Risk is determined by the specific gene mutation	High risk (C)	By 5 years of age
	Highest risk (D)	ASAP within the first year of life
Criteria for delaying prophylactic thyroidectomy: normal annual serum calcitonin, normal annual neck ultrasound, family history of less aggressive MTC		

Table 2: MEN and Medullary Thyroid Cancer

Quick Hits

  - Radioactive Iodine ablation does not work for MTC
  - Avoid injuring the Superior Laryngeal Nerve by ligation close to the superior pole of the thyroid
  - MC symptom of elevated calcitonin is diarrhea

02 THYROID

03 PARATHYROID

High Yield Anatomy and Physiology

- What is the relationship of the parathyroid glands and the recurrent laryngeal nerve?
  - Superior parathyroids are posterior and lateral to RLN
    - Originate from 4th pharyngeal pouch
  - Inferior parathyroids are anterior and medial to RLN
    - Originate from 3rd pharyngeal pouch
    - Inferior glands more variable
    - Thymus also migrates with 3rd pharyngeal pouch
  - Inferior thyroid artery provides blood supply to all 4 glands in 80% of cases

- What cells release parathyroid hormone (PTH), and what is the stimulus?
  - PTH released from chief cells in parathyroid in response to low Ca levels

- What cells release calcitonin and what is the stimulus?
  - Calcitonin is released from parafollicular c-cells in the thyroid in response to high calcium

- What are the actions of PTH on bone and in the kidney?
  - Bone -- Stimulates osteoclasts for resorption of Ca and phosphate
  - Kidneys – Stimulates resorption of Ca, inhibits resorption of phosphate and bicarb, Stimulates conversion of 25(OH)D3 to 1,25(OH)2D3 via 1-alpha hydroxylase (phosphate trashing hormone)

- How does Vit D (1,25OH2D3) increase serum Ca?
  - Stimulates absorption of Ca and Phosphate in gut

- How does Calcitonin decrease serum Ca in the bone and the kidney?
  - Bone -- Inhibits osteoclast bone resorption
  - Kidney – Inhibits resorption of Ca and phosphate

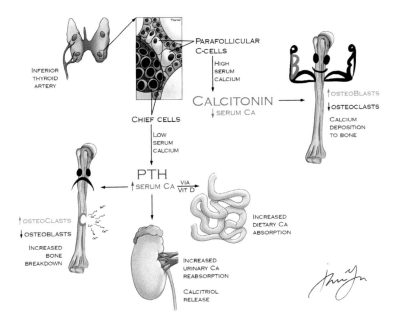

Figure 1: Parathyroid Hormone Physiology

- What is the most common cause of hypercalcemia in the outpatient and inpatient setting?
  - Outpatient = primary hyperparathyroidism
  - Inpatient = Malignancy

- What is the mechanism of hypercalcemia due to malignancy?
  - MCC hypercalcemia 2/2 malignancy is production of PTH related protein (e.g. Squamous cell lung CA, Breast CA)
  - Lytic bone lesions are less common malignant cause of hypercalcemia

- What is the treatment of a hypercalcemic crisis?
  - Treat with fluids (normal saline around 300ml/hr) and lasix once patient is euvolemic. Initially just saline. Why not LR?
  - LR has calcium

- What. are the most common causes of primary

hyperparathyroidism?

- o Adenoma (80-90%; 2-5% have double adenoma)
- o Hyperplasia (10-15%)
- o Parathyroid CA (<1%), MEN 1 and 2A

- What are the laboratory tests used to diagnose hyperparathyroidism?
  - o Increased Ca (24-hour collection), Decreased Phos (except with renal failure)
  - o Elevated serum PTH (normal 5-40 pg/dL)
  - o Chloride to Phosphate ratio >33 (Very specific)
  - o Increased Urinary Ca, Increased urinary cAMP

Chloride/Phos ratio > 33 is a reliable way to diagnose hyperparathyroidism and frequently tested.

- What studies can be used to localize an adenoma?
  - o Non-invasive – U/S, sestamibi, Single photon emission CT (SPECT), MRI
    - Best is likely sestamibi with SPECT + U/S
  - o Invasive – angiography with venous sampling for PTH gradients
    - Reserved for re-operative cases

- What is the treatment for hyperparathyroidism and who should undergo treatment?
  - o Parathyroidectomy is only long-term treatment for HPT
  - o Clear evidence that symptomatic patients should undergo surgery

- What are the indications for asymptomatic patients to undergo parathyroidectomy?
  - o Elevation of Serum Ca 1 mg/dL or more over normal value
  - o Decreased Cr Clearance (<60mL/min)
  - o T-score < -2.5

- o Poor access to care/follow-up

- o Age <50

- o Some argue all patients with HPT should get surgery

- How do you confirm adequate intraoperative resection of a parathyroid adenoma?
  - o Measure intraoperative rapid PTH assay – Need 50% drop

- How do you treat multi-gland parathyroid disease
  - o subtotal parathyroidectomy (3.5 glands) or total parathyroidectomy with reimplantation into SCM or brachioradialis

- In what patients do you see secondary hyperparathyroidism and what is the treatment?
  - o In patients with renal failure
  - o Treat with Ca/Vit D supplements, renal diet, phosphate binders

- In what patients do you see tertiary hyperparathyroidism and what is the treatment?
  - o Continued high production of PTH despite renal transplant
  - o Tx: subtotal parathyroidectomy or subtotal with auto-transplantation

- In what patients would you be concerned for parathyroid cancer and what is the treatment?
  - o Generally, have very high calcium levels, may have palpable mass.
  - o Rare cause of hyperparathyroidism
  - o Tx: En bloc resection with ipsilateral thyroid and central neck dissection
    - Recurrence/Metastasis treated with palliative surgery, calcium lowering drugs (bisphosphates/calcimimetics). Chemorads rarely effective.

Quick Hits

- A patient with high-normal range serum Ca with elevated PTH and evidence of bone loss, what is the diagnosis?
  - Normocalcemic hyperparathyroidism
  - Early form of primary HPT
  - Surgery if symptomatic

- What are the electrolyte disturbances found with hyperparathyroidism:
  - Hyperchloremic metabolic acidosis
  - d/t PTH effect on bicarb excretion in kidney
  - Hypophosphatemia
    - However, with significant renal impairment, phosphate may be elevated

- A patient with elevated PTH, elevated Ca, Low urinary Ca, what is the diagnosis and treatment?
  - Benign Familial Hypocalciuric Hypercalcemia
  - Tx? Nothing

- The inferior thyroid artery supplies parathyroid gland laterally or medially?
  - Medially

- During a neck exploration for hyperparathyroidism you find 3 normal glands and missing superior gland, where should you look next?
  - Check retroesophageal space and open carotid sheath

- During a neck exploration and you find 3 normal glands and missing inferior gland, where should you look next?
  - Check ipsilateral side of mediastinal thymus, consider intra-thyroid gland

- You find 4 normal appearing glands with elevated PTH?
  - Consider hypersecreting, supernumerary parathyroid gland most commonly located in thymus thymectomy

- Where is the most common location of a missed gland?
  - NORMAL anatomic position

- Where is the most common location of an ectopic gland?
  - Thymus

04 ESOPHAGUS

High Yield Anatomy and Physiology

- Layers of esophagus
  - Mucosa
  - Submucosa
  - Muscularis propia
  - NO SEROSA

- Esophageal blood supply
  - Cervical – Inferior thyroid artery
  - Thoracic – Vessels directly off aorta
  - Abdominal – Left gastric and inferior phrenic arteries

- Upper esophageal sphincter = Cricopharyngeus (innervated by superior laryngeal nerve)

- Killian's Triangle
  - Triangular area in the wall of the pharynx located superior to the cricopharyngeus muscle and inferior to the inferior constrictor muscles
  - Potentially weak spot where a pharyngoesophageal diverticulum (Zenker's diverticulum) is more likely to occur

Esophageal Perforation

- Can occur due to external trauma (rare), iatrogenic trauma (EGD, dilations, TE echo), increased luminal pressure (retching/Boerhaave), malignancy, chemical ingestion

- Diagnosis
  - CXR — may have any combination of pleural effusion, pneumomediastinum, subcutaneous emphysema, pneumothorax, sub diaphragmatic air. However, CXR may also be entirely normal.
  - Contrast esophagography is probably the study of choice (some may say oral contrast CT). Use water soluble first (Gastrografin) followed by dilute barium if no perforation is seen with gastrografin. *If the patient is aspiration risk, use only dilute barium.*

- o Most common site of perforation? — distal esophagus in the left posterolateral aspect 2-3cm above GE junction

- o Most common **Iatrogenic** location is at cricopharyngeus

- Treatment — Will vary based on location of injury, physiologic status of patient, damage to surrounding tissues, and underlying esophageal pathology.
  - o Resuscitate and start antibiotic for empiric coverage of Gram - rods, oral flora, anaerobes, and fungus (e.g. ampicillin, ceftriaxone, metronidazole, and fluconazole)
  - o Options include non-operative management for contained leaks, drainage alone, T-tube drainage, esophageal exclusion and diversion, esophageal stents/clips, primary repair with buttress, and esophagectomy with either immediate or delayed reconstruction
  - o Isolated cervical esophageal injury? → Open neck and place drains
  - o Thoracic perforation
    - Primary repair preferred if patient can tolerate — Left thoracotomy, debride devitalized tissue, myotomy to visualize full extend of mucosal injury, repair in 2 layers (inner absorbable, outer permanent), cover with well vascularized tissue (intercostal, omental, or latissimus flap), leak test, place NG past repair, drain chest, close. Also, consider placing enteral access.
      - Consider underlying pathology — consider esophagectomy for malignancy, caustic perforation, or burned out megaesophagus from achalasia
      - If perforation from achalasia and esophagus normal → perform contralateral myotomy
      - If severely devitalized esophagus and patient unstable — exclusion and diversion
        - o Closure of perforation, drainage, and cervical esophagostomy for proximal diversion
        - o Placing T-tube into defect and draining externally as controlled fistula
        - o J-tube enteral access for these situations

Esophageal Motility Disorders

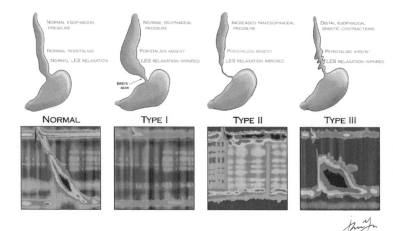

Figure 1 - Esophageal Manometry Findings

- Achalasia — Incomplete relaxation of the LES (hypertonic) WITH aperistalsis or hypotonic esophageal contractions.
  - Manometry findings, 3 Types (See Image):
    - high, or normal, LES basal pressure
    - Incomplete LES relaxation
    - Hypotonic or absent peristalsis
  - Imaging
    - Bird's beak sign on barium swallow with esophageal dilation
  - Caused by degenerative loss of nitric oxide producing inhibitory neurons within the LES, mixed etiology autoimmune, genetic, infectious
    - Causes can be idiopathic or secondary to Chagas' disease (Trypanosoma Cruzi)
    - Pseudoachalasia = achalasia caused by malignancy
  - Treatment: Minimally invasive Heller myotomy with partial fundoplication (6 cm on esophagus, 2 cm onto stomach)

- While endoscopic therapies are available (Pneumatic dilation, Botulinum toxin injection), these are less effective and increase the rate of later surgical complication, thus should be avoided for those that are good surgical candidates.

- If they perforate during a dilation make sure you do the myotomy after repairing the esophagus

- Isolated hypertensive LES
  - Manometry findings:
    - High basal LES pressure
    - Complete LES relaxation
    - Normal peristalsis
  - Tx: Ca channel blockers, nitrates, Heller

- Diffuse esophageal spasm
  - Manometry findings
    - Normal LES pressure and relaxation
    - High amplitude, <u>uncoordinated</u> esophageal contractions (>30mmHg simultaneous contractions is >10% of swallows)
  - Tx: Ca channel blockers, nitrates. Surgery is less effective. Needs long segment myotomy in extreme cases.

- Nutcracker esophagus
  - Manometry findings
    - Generally normal LES pressure and relaxation
    - High amplitude, <u>coordinated</u> esophageal contractions
  - Tx: Ca channel blockers, nitrates. Surgery is less effective. Needs long segment myotomy in extreme cases.

Esophageal Diverticula

- Zenker's (Cervical) Diverticulum — due to dysfunction of superior esophageal sphincter muscles causing increased intraesophageal pressure
  - False pulsion diverticulum

- Division of upper esophageal sphincter is key to preventing continued symptoms, recurrence, and post operative fistula

    - Diverticulum >3cm — Endoscopic division of upper esophageal sphincter, creating a common lumen between diverticulum and esophagus is an effective option

    - For diverticulum <3cm — need open myotomy (via left neck incision) with or without diverticulectomy (resection or suspension of diverticula)

- Epiphrenic esophageal diverticula
    - Pulsion diverticulum

    - Associated with esophageal motility disorders

    - Treatment: Diverticulectomy and treatment of underlying motility disorder (generally requires Heller myotomy)

- Thoracic, mid-esophageal, diverticula
    - Different in that it is often a TRACTION diverticula (True diverticula), commonly associated with adjacent inflammatory conditions (e.g. tuberculosis, malignancy), although can also be pulsion caused by mobility disorder

    - If symptomatic — VATS diverticulectomy and myotomy

Barrett's Esophagus

Definition: Intestinal metaplasia of the lower esophagus (Squamous → Columnar)

- Mucosal reaction to lower esophageal injury due to reflux of gastric acid.

- 30-60x increased risk of esophageal adenocarcinoma

- What is Surveillance?
    - EGD annually with biopsies → if 2 consecutive years negative for dysplasia → EGD every 3 years

    - 4 quadrant biopsies every 1-2cm of involved segment

        - Low-grade dysplasia on biopsy? → repeat endoscopy with biopsy in 6 months

- High-grade dysplasia (HGD) on biopsy? → repeat biopsy and confirm with expert GI pathologist → endoscopic mucosal resection (EMR) if HGD confirmed
  o Answer used to be Esophagectomy — however, the rate of progression to invasive cancer may be lower than originally thought.

Esophageal and Esophagogastric Junction Cancer

- Histologically classified as Squamous Cell Cancer (SCC) or Adenocarcinoma
  o both are more common in men
  o SCC more common in Asia and Eastern Europe
  o Adenocarcinoma is more common in N. American and W. Europe
  o Tobacco and ETOH strong risk factors for SCC
  o Obesity, GERD, Barretts are major risk factors for Adenocarcinoma
  o Often advanced stage at time of diagnosis

- Work-up
  o H&P, labs, endoscopy with biopsy (+bronch if tumor above carina), CT chest/abdomen.
    - EUS with FNA of suspicious nodes **and PET/CT** also recommended for staging

- Staging Pearls
  o T Stage
    - T1
    - 1a — Invades lamina propria or muscularis mucosa
    - 1b — Invades submucosa (important distinction because rich submucosal lymphatic system
  - T2 — Invades muscularis propria
  - T3 — Invades adventitia (remember, no serosa)
  - T4 — Invades surrounding structures

- 4a - Resectable (invades pleura, pericardium, diaphragm)
- 4b - Unresectable (invades aorta, vertebrae, trachea)
- N Stage
  - N1 — Involves 1-2 nodes
  - N2 — Involves 3-6 nodes
  - N3 — 7 or more nodes
- M1 - distant metastasis
- Grade is also important for management decisions (e.g. EMR vs esophagectomy for small superficial lesions, neoadjuvant vs surgery first, etc.)
- Stage
  - I — T1, N0, M0
  - II — Up to T3, N0, M0 or T2, N1, M0
  - III — Up to T4, N3, M0
  - IV — Distant mets

- Management
  - Randomized trials have shown preoperative chemoradiation (CROSS study) and perioperative chemotherapy (MAGIC Trial) improves survival in patient with resectable esophageal and esophagogastric CA
  - Thoracic esophageal CA >5cm from cricopharyngeus, abdominal esophageal CA, and EGJ CA → should be considered for esophagectomy for resectable lesions
  - Cervical or cervicothroacic esophageal CA <5cm for cricopharyngeus → Definitive chemoradiation, No esophagectomy
  - NCCN Recommendations
    - HGD, Tis or select T1a tumors (<2cm and well to moderate differentiation with no e/o lymph node metastasis) → Endoscopic resection +/- ablation
    - T1b, N0 tumors → Esophagectomy (Some say treat select T1b (small superficial T1b without NVI with EMR/ablation, but controversial)

- young patients, and those with high grade T1 lesions may be candidates for neoadjuvant chemoradiation
- T2 or greater or any N+ → Neoadjuvant chemoradiation followed by esophagectomy if resectable
- Unresectable (T4b or M1) → Definitive chemoradiation

o Fluorouracil or Taxane based therapy for perioperative and definitive chemo

o Surgical approaches

- Transthoracic Esophagectomy
  - Ivor-Lewis esophagectomy — Laparotomy and right thoracotomy with upper thoracic esophagogastric anastomosis — good for distal tumors
    - o Stomach mobilized and used as conduit, preservation of right gastric and right gastroepiploic artery
  - McKeown esophagectomy is similar except anastomosis made higher (cervical anastomosis) — better for more proximal lesions
- Transhiatal Esophagectomy
  - Laparotomy and left cervical incision with cervical anastomosis
    - o Advantages: Avoid morbidity of thoracotomy, leak with cervical anastomosis better tolerated than thoracic leak
    - o Disadvantages: Potentially smaller lymph node harvest, Large mid thoracic level tumors may be difficult to mobilize
    - o Equal long term survival as Transthoracic approach
- Minimally invasive techniques are also options in experienced hands (thoracoscopic, laparoscopic, and robotic mobilization)

- Patient had previous gastric resection → Colon interposition conduit

o Adjuvant therapy

- IN GENERAL (Some Caveats, but for Boards):

  - SCC does not need adjuvant therapy if R0 resection (regardless of nodal status)

  - Adenocarcinoma generally get adjuvant chemo, except when:

    o T1, N0 and R0 resection and did NOT receive neoadjuvant therapy

Quick Hits

o Anatomic areas of esophageal narrowing? — at the cricopharyngeus muscle, aortic arch, left mainstem bronchus, LES

- Esophagus most vulnerable to injury at these sites

o Primary blood supply to gastric conduit after esophagectomy?

- Right gastroepiploic

o Patient with dysphagia and you note skin thickening on palms/soles?

- Tylosis — Autosomal dominant condition linked to chromosome 17q25 associated with palmoplantar keratoma

- 40-90% risk of SCC of esophagus by age 70 — annual Upper GI starting at age 20

o SCC of head and neck, esophagus, and pancytopenia

- Fanconi Anemia (not syndrome)

o Patient with locally advanced esophageal cancer is undergoing neoadjuvant chemoradiation, has severe dysphagia and is malnourished → what feeding tube are you going to place?

- Jejunal feeding tube — NO G-TUBE OR PEG — Preserve gastric conduit

- o Dysphagia with well circumscribed, ovoid 6cm mass on barium swallow in wall of mid esophagus?
  - Esophageal leiomyoma — Most common benign tumor of esophagus
  - Treatment: For symptomatic tumors or tumors >5cm → Enucleation via VATS or thoracotomy (Right sided approach for mid esophageal lesions, Left sided approach for distal lesions)
  - **DO NOT Biopsy** — Creates mucosal scarring and makes enucleation more dangerous/difficult
- o Patient with longstanding GERD and now with dysphagia. EGD demonstrates a narrowed ring of mucosal just above the GE junction.
  - Schatzki's ring, found at the squamocolumnar junction
    - Dilation and PPI, NO RESECTION
- o Approaches to esophagus by level
  - Cervical – Left neck
  - Mid thoracic – Right chest
  - Distal – Left chest

05 STOMACH

High Yield Anatomy

- What are the types of hiatal hernias?
  - Type 1 (> 90%) - sliding
  - Type 2 - purely paraesophageal (needs repair)
  - Type 3 - combined sliding and paraesophageal (needs repair)
  - Type 4 - entire stomach in the chest plus another organ, most commonly colon (needs repair)

- What are the types of gastric ulcers?

Type	Mechanism	Location	Diagram
I	M	Lesser curve	
II	A	Lesser curve + duodenal (2 ulcers)	
III	A	Pre-pyloric	
IV	M	Proximal lesser curve (cardia)	
V	NSAIDs	Diffuse	

M = decreased mucosal protection
A = increased acid production

Table 1 – Types of gastric ulcers

- What is the Siewert-Stein Classification of esophago-gastric junction (EGJ) tumors
  - Type I — distal part of the esophagus (located between 1-5 cm above the anatomic EGJ)
  - Type II — cardia (within 1 cm above and 2 cm below the EGJ)
  - Type III — subcardial stomach (2-5 cm below EGJ)

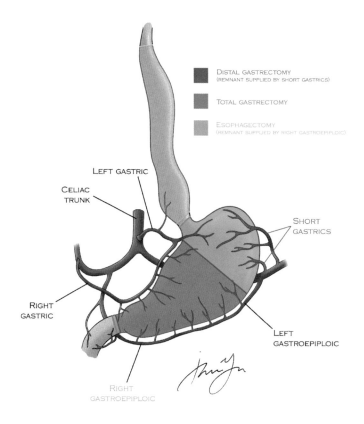

Figure 1 – Vascular anatomy of the stomach

Gastric Volvulus

o What are the features?

- Often associated with paraesophageal hernias
- High morbidity and mortality

o What are the three types?

- Organoaxial (most common) — rotation along the axis of the stomach from the GE junction to the pylorus
- Mesoaxial (less common) — rotation along short axis of stomach bisecting the lesser and greater curvature
- Combined

o How are these treated?

- Typically with emergent surgery → hernia repair, gastropexy, partial gastrectomy if devitalized
- Endoscopic decompression can be attempted in frail (risk of perforation) with double PEG tubes

Gastroesophageal reflux disease (GERD)

o What are the alarm symptoms?

- Dysphagia, odynophagia, weight loss, anemia, GI bleeding
- Concern for malignancy → upper endoscopy

o How is GERD medically managed?

- Lifestyle modification: weight loss, elevate head of bed, avoid aggravating foods
- Proton pump inhibitors (PPI)
  - If no improvement over several weeks on PPI → need EGD
- What are the indications for surgical evaluation?
  - Failure of medical management
  - Desire to avoid lifelong PPI
  - Extra-esophageal manifestations - asthma, hoarseness, cough, chest pain, aspiration

> If atypical symptoms and GI surgical history, think bile reflux. Work up with impedance probe and management is usually Roux-en-Y reconstruction.

o What is the pre-operative work up?

- Barium swallow
- Upper endoscopy
- Ambulatory pH testing
- Esophageal manometry to rule out underlying motility disorder (can't do full Nissen if dysmotility)

o What are the components of 24-hour esophageal pH monitoring?

- Percent total time pH<4
- Percent upright time pH<4
- Percent supine time pH<4
- Number of reflux episodes
- Number of reflux episodes ≥ 5 min
- Longest reflux episode (minutes)
- Demeester score > 14.72 = reflux

o Operative management

- What are the overall surgical goals?
    - Restoration of normal anatomic position of the stomach and GE junction
    - Recreation of anti-reflux valve
    - Any hiatal hernia must be completely reduced → requires mediastinal dissection to ensure adequate esophageal mobilization
    - Any defect in diaphragmatic crura must be adequately closed
    - Complete mobilization of the fundus
    - 2 cm long "floppy" fundoplication performed over large (54F) bougie

- ○ Partial fundoplication/alternates to 360° Nissen
  - • Dor (anterior 180–200°)
  - • Toupet (posterior 270°)
  - • Thal (270° anterior)
  - • Belsey (270° anterior transthoracic)
  - • Lind (300° posterior)
  - • Hill repair
  - ○ Insufficient evidence to support one over another. Some data shows less postop dysphagia with partial wrap compared to 360° wraps, however, may have inadequate control of reflux.
- • In the OR, anesthesia is having trouble ventilating patient. What are you worried about?
  - • Capnothorax
- ○ Enlarge tear to avoid tension capnothorax
- ○ Place red rubber catheter with one end into pleural tear and other end into abdomen (equalizes pressures)
- ○ At end of procedure bring one end outside of abdomen and place to water seal while Valsalva administered
- ○ Can also needle decompress intra-operatively – be sure to prep lower chest

> High end tidal CO2 during mediastinal dissection is most likely capnothorax. May also be hypoventilation, CO2 embolus, or malignant hyperthermia.

- • What if the post op CXR shows a 2 cm pneumothorax?
  - • Don't do anything, will self-resolve
- • How do you manage these patients postoperatively?
  - • Schedule anti-emetics immediately postop (avoid nausea/retching)
  - • Soft diet for a few weeks
  - • Avoid meat, raw vegetables, bread, carbonated beverages for 4-6 weeks

- What is the management of postop dysphagia?

  - Very common

  - Severe dysphagia → esophagram

  - Dysphagia persisting past 6 weeks postop → esophagram (concern for recurrent hernia, slipped wrap) → if not present, dilation

Hiatal Hernia

- How are these diagnosed?

  - Often seen on CXR

    - Barium swallow, CT chest, and EGD and are used in various combinations depending on individual patient presentation.

- What is the management?

  - Repair of type I in the absence of reflux disease is not indicated → same operative indications as for GERD

  - All symptomatic paraesophageal hernias (types 2-4) should be repaired, especially those with obstructive symptoms or those that have volvulized

> Type I = sliding, Type II = paraesophageal, Type III – both, Type IV = another organ

  - Asymptomatic paraesophageal hernias should be repaired on a routine, elective basis if the patient is a good surgical candidate

    - Watchful waiting is an option for asymptomatic or minimally symptomatic patients who are poor surgical candidates

  - Laparoscopic repair is the preferred approach, although may also be repaired via open or trans-thoracic approach

    - Hernia sac needs to be mobilized and excised (key step that decreases early recurrence)

    - Use of mesh in large (> 5-8 cm) hiatal hernia decreases short-term recurrence. However, many questions remain regarding the long-term safety.

Currently, insufficient evidence to recommend one way or the other regarding routine use of mesh reinforcement, but probably reasonable with large defects.

- Permanent suture to close crura
- Fundoplication should be performed at time of repair (same principles as when done for GERD regarding mediastinal mobilization and length of intra-abdominal esophagus needed) → Collis gastroplasty (esophageal lengthening)
    o Gastropexy or gastrostomy tube may be added if needed if not bad enough to need extra length

Gastroduodenal Ulcer Disease
  o What is the association with H. pylori?
  - H. pylori is found in 75% of gastric ulcer disease and 95% of duodenal ulcer patients
  - What is the treatment?
    - Triple therapy
      o PPI
      o Clarithromycin
      o Amoxicillin or metronidazole
  o Gastroduodenal Ulcers
  - What are the management principles for bleeding gastric and duodenal ulcers?
    - First step is typical resuscitative measures and early endoscopy, NG tube placement
      o Rapid upper endoscopy is usually diagnostic and therapeutic
        - Endoscopic clips, thermal coagulation, injection of vasoactive or sclerosing agent
      o Endoscopic interventions are 90% effective for controlling initial bleeding

- o What is the risk of rebleeding?
    - • Actively bleeding pulsatile vessel — up to 80%
    - • Visible vessel — up to 50%
    - • Adherent clot — 15-25%
    - • Clean base — <5%
- Gastric Ulcer
  - • What is important in treating gastric ulcers?
    - o Biopsy ulcer to evaluate for malignancy as well as obtain antral biopsies to test for H. pylori.
      - • MC cause of gastric bleeding = H. pylori and NSAIDs
      - • Underlying malignancy present in approximately 5% of gastric ulcers
  - • What do you do if patient rebleeds after 1st endoscopic intervention?
    - o Repeat endoscopy (angiography also an option)
    - o Once bleeding is controlled, etiology has to be identified and treated
      - • Stop NSAIDS, tobacco cessation, PPI, H. Pylori treatment, etc.
  - • When do you operate?
    - o For bleeding that cannot be controlled endoscopically or hemorrhagic shock → midline laparotomy, anterior gastrotomy, oversew bleeding area, biopsy, and close gastrotomy
- Duodenal Ulcer
  - • What is the management of a bleeding duodenal ulcer?
    - o Initial management same as any upper GI bleed → resuscitate, NG tube, rapid EGD for diagnosis/treatment

- Endoscopy is 1st and 2nd line (like gastric ulcers) → possibly angiography → surgery reserved for uncontrolled bleeding with above and hemodynamic instability

- What operation?

  - Longitudinal anterior duodenotomy, control bleeding with sutures placed superior and inferior to ulcer taking care to avoid CBD (can ligate GDA above duodenum if bleeding continues) → approximate ulcer crater → close duodenotomy transversely

- How do you treat perforated ulcers?

  - Initiate fluid resuscitation, NG decompression, acid suppression, and antibiotics for empiric coverage of gram-negative rods, oral flora, anaerobes, and fungus (e.g. ampicillin, ceftriaxone, metronidazole, <u>fluconazole</u>)

  - Omental patch repair

    - May be performed open or laparoscopically

    - Close perforation with seromuscular bite if able to approximate and then secure tongue of omentum over site of perforation with 3-4 sutures

 A small amount of free air and stable patient may have a contained perforation that does not require OR. However, not a common exam scenario.

- If patient undergoing operation for complication of gastroduodenal ulcer disease and has hx of treatment with PPI and/or eradication of h. pylori (i.e. refractory ulcer disease), what else should you consider?

  - Acid reducing procedure

    - Truncal vagotomy and pyloroplasty

    - Highly selective vagotomy (HSV) - Preserves motor innervation to pylorus, eliminating need for drainage procedure

- o Vagotomy and antrectomy — Higher morbidity (2/2 need for Bilroth reconstruction) than vagotomy and pyloroplasty or HSV, therefore, reserved for stable patients with anatomic indications (large antral ulcers, pyloric scarring)

 Marginal ulcer after bariatric surgery perforation treated the same as duodenal ulcer.

Gastric Cancer

- o What are the risk factors?
  - • H. pylori, smoking, heavy ETOH intake, high salt, nitrates
- o Typically classified as intestinal type or diffuse type (Lauren Classification)
- o Most are sporadic, 5-10% familial component, 3-5% inherited syndrome
  - • Hereditary diffuse gastric cancer
    - • Autosomal dominant disorder 2/2 germline mutation in *CDH1*
    - • How do you treat these patients?
      - o Prophylactic gastrectomy recommended between age 18-40 for *CDH1* carriers
    - • Women with *CDH1* are at increased risk of breast CA similar to BRCA patients
  - • What are other hereditary syndromes with increased risk of gastric CA?
    - • Lynch syndrome (DNA mismatch genes)
    - • Juvenile polyposis syndrome (SMAD4)
    - • Peutz-Jehgers Syndrome
    - • Familial adenomatous polyposis (APC gene on 5q21)
- o How do you stage these?
  - • Routine labs, CT chest/abdomen/pelvis, EUS with FNA, PET/CT

o What is the role of staging laparoscopy?

- NCCN recommends laparoscopic staging with peritoneal washing for clinical stage > T1b tumors if chemoradiation or surgery being considered (not needed if known metastasis and undergoing definitive chemoradiation or palliative options)

  - Staging Pearls —

    o T stage

      - T1

        - T1a invades lamina propria or muscularis mucosa

        - T1b invades submucosa

      - T2 invades muscularis propria

      - T3 invades subserosa

      - T4 invades through serosa or into adjacent structures

    o N status

      - N1 involves 1-2 nodes

      - N2 involves 3-6 nodes

      - N3 involves 7 or more nodes

Staging similar to esophageal cancer, but esophagus has no serosa.

o What is unresectable disease?

- Peritoneal involvement, distal metastases, root of mesentery involvement or para-aortic nodal disease confirmed by biopsy, encasement of major vascular structure (excluding splenic vessels)

o Who gets neoadjuvant therapy?

- cT2 or higher and any N

Similar to esophageal and rectal cancer

o What are the surgical principles?

- Resection with at least 4 cm margins and lymph node harvest of at least 15

    - Type of resection (total vs subtotal gastrectomy) and extent of lymph node dissection (D1 vs D2) is somewhat controversial

    - Subtotal gastrectomy is preferred for distal lesions (Siewert III)

    - Proximal tumors (Siewert II) will generally need total gastrectomy with esophagojejunostomy, distal portion of esophagus may need to be resected for adequate margins

    - Tumors crossing GE junction are classified and treated as esophageal cancer

- NO prophylactic splenectomy (only if spleen or hilum grossly involved with tumor)

- T4 tumors require en bloc resection of involved structures

- What are the types of lymph node dissection?

    - D1 dissection = removal of N1 nodes (perigastric nodes along greater/lesser curve, stations 1-6)

    - D2 dissection = removal of N1 and N2 nodes (nodes along left gastric, common hepatic, celiac and splenic arteries, stations 7-11)

    - Gastrectomy with D2 dissection is the standard in Asia, however, Western studies have failed to demonstrate survival benefit of D2 dissection over D1 dissection, and D2 dissection may be associated with increased morbidity/mortality → current NCCN recommendation is for R0 resection with at least D1 or modified D2 lymph node dissection

        o R0 = negative microscopic margin

        o R1 = negative gross margin, positive microscopic margin

        o R2 = positive gross margin

o When is adjuvant therapy recommended?

- Adjuvant 5-fluorouracil for T3, T4, or node positive disease following R0 resection

Post Gastrectomy Syndromes

o What is retained antrum syndrome?

- Retained antral tissue within duodenal stump after gastric resection

  - G cells bathed in alkaline fluid → continuous gastrin release → acid production in proximal stomach remnant and ulceration

Check gastrin levels to rule out a gastrin-secreting tumor.

- Treatment = PPI; vagotomy and resection of retained antrum

o What is dumping syndrome?

- Tachycardia, diaphoresis, dizziness, flushing

- Early dumping syndrome (20-30 min after meal)

  - Occurs due to abrupt hyperosmolar load to small intestine

- Late dumping syndrome (1-4 hours after meal)

  - Due to rapid carbohydrate load to small intestine resulting in large insulin surge and rebound hypoglycemia

- Majority managed with small meals, no sugary drinks → for refractory dumping syndrome try octreotide

o What is alkaline reflux gastritis?

- After Bilroth I and Bilroth II reconstructions

- Diagnosis = impedance studies

- What is medical management?

  - Pro kinetic agents, bile acid binding resins

- What is surgical management?

  - Conversion to RNY

At least 50 cm for Roux limb will avoid recurrent bile reflux.

- What is the Braun enterostomy?

    o Anastomosis between afferent and efferent limb

o What is afferent limb syndrome?

  • Acute or chronic obstruction of afferent jejunal limb following Bilroth II reconstruction

  • Increased luminal pressure of afferent limb can result in what symptoms?

    • Obstructive jaundice, cholangitis, pancreatitis from back pressure up biliopancreatic system

    • Duodenal stump blow out

    • Bacterial overgrowth in afferent limb → bacteria deconjugate bile acids → steatorrhea, malnutrition, and vitamin B-12 deficiency leading to megaloblastic anemia.

  • Treatment = conversion to Roux-en-Y or Bilroth I; bacterial overgrowth can be managed first with antibiotics (high relapse rate though)

 If B2 patient presents with bowel obstruction, no NGT and decompression → emergent surgery. Similar to bypass patients with internal hernia.

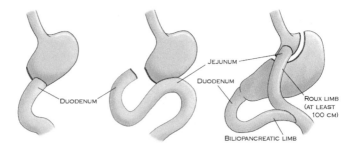

COMPLICATIONS		
BILLROTH I	**BILLROTH II**	**ROUX-EN-Y**
MARGINAL ULCER	MARGINAL ULCER	MARGINAL ULCER
RETAINED ANTRAL TISSUE	RETAINED ANTRAL TISSUE	
BILE REFLUX	BILE REFLUX	
	BLIND LOOP SYNDROME	BLIND LOOP SYNDROME
	AFFERENT LOOP OBSTRUCTION	AFFERENT LOOP OBSTRUCTION
	DUODENAL STUMP BLOWOUT	
	DUMPING SYNDROME	

Figure 2 – Gastric reconstruction options with associated complications

Quick Hits

- What do you do if you need more esophageal length during paraesophageal hernia repair?
  - o Collis gastroplasty

- Unable to swallow secretions after Nissen, what's the problem and management?
  - o Wrap too tight, return to OR

- Types of ulcer associated with increased acid output?
  - o Type II and III

- Types of ulcer associated with decreased mucosal protection?
  - o Type I and IV

- Hiatal hernia discovered at time of sleeve gastrectomy. What do you do?
  - o Repair

- Patient with history of antrectomy and Bilroth II reconstruction in distant past presents with intermittent abdominal pain and

distention which is relieved after bilious emesis, megaloblastic anemia on laboratory work up. What is this?
○ Afferent limb syndrome

• What is the diagnosis for a patient with multiple duodenal ulcers and gastrin levels >1000 pg/ml?
○ Zollinger Ellison syndrome

• Gastric mass with biopsy showing expansion of the marginal zone compartment with development of sheets of neoplastic small lymphoid cells. Diagnosis and treatment?
○ Maltoma

○ Treatment = antibiotics (triple therapy for H. pylori)

  • Will typically regress once H. pylori is eradicated

06 SPLEEN

High Yield Anatomy/Physiology

- Main Ligaments (there are more minor ligaments, but these are the most surgically important)
  - Gastrosplenic → contains short gastrics
  - Splenorenal → contains splenic vessels and tail of pancreas
  - Splenocolic
  - Splenophrenic

- Spleen functions:
  - Store platelets, filter senescent erythrocytes, re-energize erythrocytes through "pitting", immune function (largest concentration of lymphoid tissue in the body)
    - Pitting = removal of intracellular products
  - Opsonization: Tuftsin and Properdin

- Red pulp — Filters RBCs — Most of the spleen — Thin walled sinusoids separated by cords containing red cells

- White pulp — Immune functions
  - Lymphoid follicles — B-cells
  - Periarterial lymphatic sheath (PALS) — T-cells

- Peripheral blood smear suggesting absent/damaged spleen:
  - Howell-Jolly body = Nuclear remnants (most reliable finding)
  - Pappenheimer body = Iron deposits
  - Target cell = Immature RBC
  - Heinz body = Intracellular denatured hemoglobin
  - Spur cell = Deformed membrane
  - What if you don't see these post-splenectomy
    - Accessory spleen

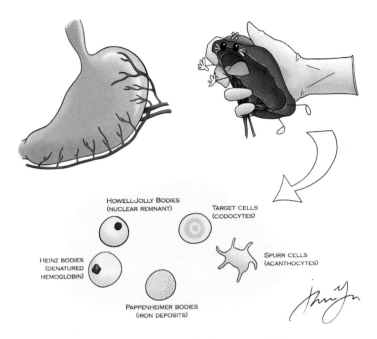

Figure 1 - Figure 1 - Hematologic Consequence of Splenectomy

Indications for splenectomy

- Unstable trauma patients

- Hematologic disorders: MC ITP and spherocytosis

- Splenic abscess

- Symptomatic cysts

- Primary malignancies (mainly non-Hodgkins lymphomas)

Splenic Trauma

- Can be secondary to iatrogenic trauma from splenic capsular tear with over vigorous retraction during foregut or colon procedures

- Penetrating trauma → splenectomy

- Blunt injury → selective non-operative management

○ Patient must be hemodynamically stable without peritonitis → Otherwise emergent laparotomy and splenectomy

○ Nonoperative management includes in-hospital or ICU monitoring, serial abdominal examinations, serial hematocrit measurements, and a period of immobility (bed rest/post-discharge restricted activity)

○ Angiographic intervention should be considered for:

• AAST grade >III injuries (subcapsular hematoma >50% or expanding; ruptured subcapsular hematoma; laceration >3cm or involving trabecular vessels)

• Presence of contrast blush

• Moderate hemoperitoneum

• Any signs of ongoing splenic bleeding

Hematologic Disorders

• Idiopathic thrombocytopenia purpura (ITP)

○ Thought to be caused by autoantibodies to glycoproteins IIb/IIIa and Ia/IIa

○ Initial management is medical → Steroids, IVIG

○ Splenectomy for medically refractory cases or for recurrence (avoids need for longstanding steroids)

• Patients who have a good response to steroids → predictive of a favorable response after splenectomy

○ When do you transfuse platelets?

• Only for intraoperative bleeding → give after ligating splenic artery if possible (prevents consumption of transfused platelets)

• Hereditary Spherocytosis

○ Presentation: anemia, splenomegaly

○ Autosomal dominant defect in cell membrane protein (spectrin) → RBC less deformable → culled by spleen

○ Splenectomy recommended for symptomatic patients older than 6 years old (want them to develop immune function prior to splenectomy)

- Typically, will require cholecystectomy at time of surgery as well (check for gallstones – hemolysis produces bilirubin stones)

- Pyruvate Kinase Deficiency — Congenital hemolytic anemia caused by impaired glucose metabolism – splenectomy reduces transfusion requirements

- Hemoglobinopathies — Sickle cell disease, thalasemias — Rare indication for splenectomy

Splenic abscess

- Causes: IV drug use, endocarditis, secondary infection of traumatic pseudocyst, sickle cell disease

- Unilocular with thick wall in stable patient → percutaneous drainage

- Multi-locular, thin walled → suspect echinoccocal abscess → Splenectomy

Splenic lesions

- Splenic cyst
  - Well defined hypodense lesion without an enhancing rim
  - Two types
    - True cysts: congenital, parasitic (echinococcus), or neoplastic
    - False cysts: post traumatic pseudocyst
  - Leave alone if asymptomatic (serology and imaging characteristics can typically rule out parasitic cyst or malignancy)
  - Large cysts (>5cm) or symptomatic → Consider laparoscopic cyst excision or fenestration

- Hemangioma = MC splenic tumor → splenectomy if symptomatic

- Angiosarcoma = primary malignant tumor of spleen
  - Associated with vinyl chloride and thorium dioxide exposure

- o Aggressive, high mortality
- o Splenectomy if caught in time

- Non-Hodgkins lymphoma
  - o MC CLL → Splenectomy for anemia/thrombocytopenia

Splenic artery aneurysm

- MC visceral artery aneurysm, more common in women

- When to treat?
  - o >2cm
  - o All pregnant women or women of childbearing age, regardless of size (As high as 70% rupture risk during pregnancy

- Treatment → Usually endovascular coil embolization of the aneurysm or placement of covered stent
  - o Very distal aneurysms may require splenectomy
  - o Tradition open or laparoscopic splenic artery ligation also acceptable options

Post splenectomy infection

- Decreased IgM and IgG leads to increased susceptibility to encapsulated organisms (S. pneumoniae, N. meningitidis, H. influenza)
  - o Timing of vaccination?
    - 2 weeks prior to elective splenectomy or prior to hospital discharge following emergent splenectomy (or 2 weeks post-op if reliable follow-up)

- OPSI risk is higher in children — especially in hematologic disease (Beta thalassemia)

- If suspicion of OPSI → Broad spectrum antibiotics immediately! — Don't wait for cultures

- Prophylactic antibiotics?
  - o Consider for children <10 years old
  - o Definitely not in adults

Quick Hits

- Patient s/p splenectomy for ITP with persistent thrombocytopenia. Periepheral smear with Howel-jolly bodies?
  - Accessory spleen
  - Diagnose with imaging: radionuclide spleen scan (tagged RBC scan)
  - MC location: splenic hilum

- MC organism associated with OPSI?
  - S. pneumo

- Abdominal pain and CT with spleen in RLQ, abdominal U/S shows no flow in splenic vein. Diagnosis?
  - Wandering spleen
    - Caused by failure of fusion of dorsal mesogastrium, leading to lack of splenic ligaments
    - Risk of splenic torsion and infarction
  - Treatment?
    - Splenectomy if splenic infarction, otherwise splenopexy

- MC source of post splenectomy bleeding?
  - Short gastrics

- Patient with abdominal pain following splenectomy. CT shows large, low attenuation, contained fluid collection in surgical bed/lesser sac. Diagnosis?
  - Pancreatic leak — tail of pancreas at risk during splenectomy
  - Treatment?
    - Percutaneous drain

- Patient with fever, hemolytic anemia, renal failure, purpura, neurologic changes. Diagnosis and management?
  - Thrombotic thrombocytopenic purpura (TTP)
  - FAT-RN mnemonic (Fever, Anemia, Thrombocytopenia, Renal, Neurological)
  - Caused by defective ADAMTS13 metalloproteinase (vWF cleaving protein) → Platelet aggregation in microvasculature
  - Treatment = Plasmapheresis

07 HEPATOBILIARY

PART ONE

High Yield Anatomy

- What structures are in the portal triad?
  - Common bile duct
  - Proper hepatic artery (medial)
  - Portal vein (posterior)
  - Runs in hepatoduodenal ligament

- What separates the right and left lobes of the liver?
  - Cantlie's Line (line between gallbladder fossa and IVC)

- What numbers correspond to the anatomic liver segments?
  - I = caudate lobe
  - II-III = left lateral segments
  - IV = left inferior anteromedial
  - V = right inferior anteromedial
  - VI-VII = right posterior lateral
  - VIII = right superior anteromedial

- What is the venous drainage?
  - 3 hepatic veins → drain into IVC
  - Medial and left hepatic vein usually merge before draining into IVC

- What are the most common aberrant vascular anatomy?
  - Replaced right hepatic – most commonly off the SMA, travels behind pancreas and CBD
  - Replaced left hepatic – most commonly off the left gastric, travels in gastrohepatic ligament

> During foregut surgery, take care not to ligate a replaced left traveling in the gastrohepatic ligament.

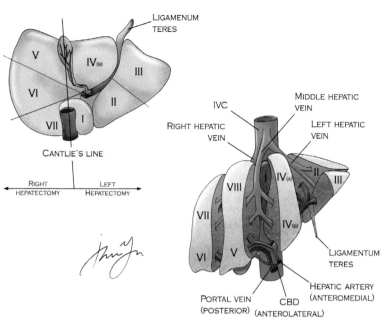

Figure 1 – Segmental anatomy of the liver

Benign Biliary Disease

- o What is the management of asymptomatic gallstones?
  - • Observation
- o What about uncomplicated symptomatic cholelithiasis?
  - • Elective cholecystectomy
- o How do you manage symptomatic cholelithiasis in pregnancy?
  - • Higher rates of spontaneous abortion with non-operative management
  - • Laparoscopic cholecystectomy during the second trimester
    - • Place ports via open Hassan technique
    - • Keep pneumoperitoneum as low as possible
    - • Place bump under right side to offload cava
- o How do you manage acute cholecystitis?
  - • Early cholecystectomy if surgically fit

There is no benefit to waiting or "cooling off" acute cholecystitis with antibiotics.

- Cholecystostomy tube if unable to tolerate surgery
    - If recovered from their critical illness → interval cholecystectomy
        - o Recurrent symptoms are common after cholecystostomy tube removal
- o What is the management of suspected choledocholithiasis?
    - Several acceptable approaches and much variability between institutions, but in general:
        - Strong suspicion (CBD stone on imaging, clinical cholangitis, bilirubin > 3, dilated CBD > 6 mm) → consider preop ERCP for duct clearance
            - o IOC and possible CBD exploration if ERCP not available
        - Moderate suspicion (abnormal liver tests other than bili, mild elevation in bili, clinical gallstone pancreatitis) → MRCP or IOC
        - Low suspicion (no biochemical or imaging suggestive of CBD stone) → no further investigation prior to cholecystectomy
    - CBD stones identified during IOC → flush + glucagon up to twice
        - If small stone and large enough cystic duct → transcystic CBD exploration using fluoroscopic guidance or choledochoscope
        - If not amenable to transcystic approach → either lap CBD exploration or postop ERCP depending on resources available and surgeon experience
    - What if you can't visualize the hepatic ducts on IOC?
        - Pull catheter back and try flushing again
        - Trendelenburg to see if change in imaging (back filling using gravity)

- Convert to open to investigate injury to hepatic duct
o Gallstone pancreatitis
  - Do you need to perform ERCP?
    - Only if clinical signs of cholangitis
    - Stone will likely pass and no improvement of outcomes with early ERCP in patients with gallstone pancreatitis alone
  - When do you perform cholecystectomy?
    - Should be done during index admission after clinical pancreatitis resolves
    - In severe cases with significant peripancreatic fluid collections → wait until fluid collections mature or regress → interval cholecystectomy at 6 weeks is acceptable, but an ERCP with sphincterotomy should be performed to reduce risk of complications during waiting period
o What is gallstone ileus?
  - Small bowel obstruction caused by a gallstone (typically at IC valve) resulting from a cholecystoenteric fistula (usually fistula to duodenum)
  - What is the Rigler triad?
    - Bowel obstruction
    - Gallstone seen in intestine
    - Pneumobilia on imaging
  - How do you treat this?
    - Primary goal: relieve the obstruction
      o Perform enterotomy proximal to obstruction and milk stone back and remove through enterotomy
    - Should you perform cholecystectomy and fistula takedown at the time of enterolithotomy?
      o No
      o A combined procedure has higher morbidity and recurrence rates are low

- o Can consider in select circumstances: patient stable and gangrenous cholecystitis present (in other words they're stable and REALLY need their gallbladder out)

 99% of the time the answer is enterotomy and milk the stone. Avoid cholecystectomy and fistula takedown.

- o What are gallbladder polyps?
  - Majority are benign hyperplastic polyps
  - Management
    - Symptomatic → cholecystectomy
    - Asymptomatic → cholecystectomy if > 10 mm in size
      - o If over 18 mm → treat as gallbladder cancer until proven otherwise
      - o Polyps over 6 mm need serial imaging or consider surgery to avoid need for surveillance

Portal Hypertension

- o What is the hepatic vein pressure gradient (HVPG)?
  - Gradient between the wedged hepatic vein pressure and the free hepatic vein pressure – requires passage of balloon catheter into hepatic vein under fluoroscopy
  - Portal hypertension defined as (HVPG) > 6 mmHg
- o What are the clinical effects of portal hypertension?
  - Portosystemic venous collaterals, ascites, hepatic encephalopathy, splenomegaly
- o What is the relationship between the site of increased portal resistance and the etiology of portal hypertension?
  - Presinusoidal → e.g. schistosomiasis
  - Sinusoidal → e.g. alcoholic cirrhosis, viral hepatitis
  - Postsinusoidal → Budd-Chiari syndrome
  - Many are mixed disorders (e.g. primary biliary cirrhosis has both presinusoidal and sinusoidal elements)

o What are the sites of collateral circulation?

- Where splanchnic venous system meets with systemic drainage

  - Distal esophagus/proximal stomach (esophageal submucosal veins to proximal gastric veins)

  - Rectum (IMV to pudendal vein)

  - Umbilicus (vestigial umbilical vein to left portal vein)

  - Retroperitoneum (mesenteric and ovarian veins)

o How do you treat it?

- Pharmacologic

  - Splanchnic vasoconstrictors in acute setting = vasopressin, octreotide

  - Non-selective beta-blockers for prophylaxis = nadolol, propranolol

- Endoscopic variceal banding

- Transjugular intrahepatic portosystemic shunt (TIPS)

  - Used for acute or recurrent variceal bleeding, refractory ascites, Budd-Chiari syndrome, or hepatic hydrothorax

o What is the management of acute esophageal variceal bleeding?

- Resuscitate, transfuse, antibiotics, intubation for airway protection

- Octreotide → endoscopic treatment → TIPS if uncontrolled (balloon tamponade as temporizing measure)

  - If rebleed after initial endoscopic control → 2nd endoscopy → consider TIPS

o What are the surgical options for portal hypertension?

- Gastroesophageal devascularization

  - Generally reserved for patients with extensive portal venous thrombosis and no portosystemic shunt options

- Esophageal transection with division and anastomosis
  - Rarely used since TIPS
- Devascularization procedures
  - Total devascularization of the greater curvature and upper 2/3rd of the lesser curvature and circumferential devascularization of the lower 7.5 cm of the esophagus
- Portosystemic shunts
  - Selective shunts (e.g. distal splenorenal or "Warren" shunt)
    - o Decompress only part of portal venous system
    - o Good for variceal bleeding but does not help ascites
  - Partial portosystemic shunts
    - o Type of side to side shunt where flow is calibrated by the size of the synthetic interposition graft placed between the portal vein and vena cava
  - Nonselective portosystemic shunts
    - o Decompress the entire portal venous system
    - o Side to side portocaval shunt is most common
    - o High rate of encephalopathy and complicate later liver transplant

Variceal bleeding → selective shunt. Ascites → nonselective shunt.

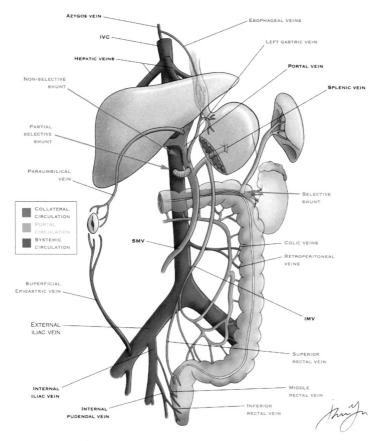

Figure 2 – Vascular anatomy of portosystemic shunts

Liver Abscess

○ What types of abscesses can be found in the liver?

- Pyogenic abscess (most common, > 80%)

    - Usually secondary to biliary tract infection (E. coli most common pathogen), GI source (diverticulitis, appendicitis)

    - Treatment = percutaneous drain and antibiotics

- Ameobic abscess

    - Typical presentation is patient with liver abscess after travel to Mexico

- Get serology
- Treatment = metronidazole, rarely needs drainage
- Echinococcal cyst
  - Hydatid cyst
  - Characteristic double walled cyst on CT
  - Check serology
  - Treatment = albendazole followed by surgical excision
    - Do not aspirate or spill → cause anaphylaxis

Quick Hits

- What hepatic vein pressure gradient is typically required for variceal rupture?
  - 12 mmHg
  - What is the definition of portal HTN?
    - 6 mmHg

- What are the components of the Child-Turcotte-Pugh score?
  - Bilirubin, albumin, prothrombin time, encephalopathy, ascites

- What are the components of the Model for End-stage Liver Disease (MELD) score?
  - Bilirubin, INR, creatinine

- What is the MELD score at which patients have a survival benefit for transplantation?
  - 15

- What is the management of umbilical hernias in a cirrhotic with ascites?
  - Ideally done in elective setting
  - Medically control ascites first
    - Control of ascites is key to reduce hernia recurrence and postoperative complications, such as wound infection, evisceration, ascites drainage, and peritonitis
    - If medical treatment of ascites doesn't work → intermittent

paracentesis, temporary peritoneal dialysis catheter or transjugular intrahepatic portosystemic shunt may be necessary

- Use mesh in the elective setting

o If patient eligible for transplant → repair hernia at time of transplant

o If complicated (incarcerated, strangulated, ruptured) → must repair urgently

- No mesh, close in layers (close peritoneum), sterile dressing

- Aggressive ascites control postop until healed

> Avoid leaving an intraperitoneal drain on the exam – patient can get hypotensive. Intermittent paracentesis is the standard.

- How do you manage symptomatic cholelithiasis in a patient with cirrhosis and ascites?
  o Medically manage until cirrhosis is compensated, then laparoscopic cholecystectomy by an experienced liver surgeon.

  o Replace clotting factors and platelets preop if necessary

PART TWO

Cystic Hepatobiliary Lesions

o What are choledochal cysts?
  - Unknown etiology but likely secondary to an anomalous biliary-pancreatic duct junction with reflux of pancreatic enzymes (long common BP duct)
  - Most are identified and treated in early childhood
  - Can cause, pain, biliary obstruction, cirrhosis
  - Carry malignant potential

○ What is the Todani classification system and treatment by type?

- I – Fusiform dilation of extrahepatic biliary tree
  - Resection with hepaticojejunostomy
- II – Saccular diverticulum of CBD
  - Excision of cyst – likely with RNY biliary enteric reconstruction
- III – Dilation of intramural duct (choledochocele)
  - Uncommon – approach transduodenally → transduodenal excision or sphincteroplasty
- IVa – Multiple dilations of intra and extra-hepatic ducts
  - Hepatic resection and biliary reconstruction
- IVb – Multiple dilations of extra-hepatic ducts
  - Excision and hepaticojejunostomy
- V – Multiple dilations of intrahepatic ducts (Caroli's)
  - Transplantation (can have one attempt at partial resection if isolated to one part of liver)

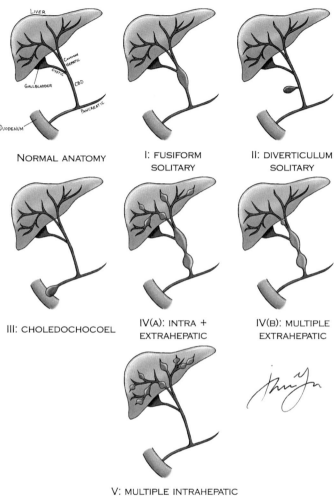

NORMAL ANATOMY

I: FUSIFORM SOLITARY

II: DIVERTICULUM SOLITARY

III: CHOLEDOCHOCOEL

IV(A): INTRA + EXTRAHEPATIC

IV(B): MULTIPLE EXTRAHEPATIC

V: MULTIPLE INTRAHEPATIC

Figure 3 – Types of choledochal cysts

○ How do you manage a simple hepatic cyst?

- No treatment if asymptomatic

- 100% recurrence rate with aspiration alone

- Laparoscopic cyst fenestration for symptomatic cysts → send capsule for pathology

- If concern for abscess, hydatid cyst, or malignancy → aspirate for cytology

Hepatobiliary Tumors

   o What are the characteristics of a hepatic hemangioma?

- Most common liver tumor, male predominance, equal distribution in liver
- Congenital vascular malformations, generally asymptomatic
  - Can cause pain, compressive symptoms
  - Rarely hemorrhage, inflammation, or coagulopathy
  - Kasabach-Merritt Syndrome = hemangioma + consumptive coagulopathy
- Imaging
  - CT: hypodense pre-contrast; peripheral → central enhancement in the arterial phase; persistent contrast on delayed series
  - MRI: hypointense on T1; hyperintense on T2
- Treatment
  - Asymptomatic → observation (regardless of size, no risk of rupture)
  - Symptomatic → resection

   o Focal Nodular Hyperplasia

- 2nd most common liver tumor, women 30-50 years old
- Completely benign, usually asymptomatic
- Imaging
  - CT: well demarcated; rapid arterial enhancement with central stellate scar
  - MRI: hypointense with central scar on T1; isointense with hyperintense scar on T2
- Treatment
  - Nothing – no malignant potential, no bleeding risk

o Adenoma

- Rare, associated with OCP and androgen steroid use
- Malignant transformation in 10%
- Risk of rupture increases with size → 30% risk of spontaneous bleeding with tumors > 5 cm
- Can present with pain, abdominal fullness, abnormal LFTs, or bleeding from rupture
- Imaging
  - CT: arterial enhancement with washout on portal phase; smooth surface with tumor capsule; no central scar
  - MRI: mildly hyperintense on T1 and T2
- Treatment
  - Small lesions → discontinue OCPs and it may regress
  - Larger lesions (> 4 cm) or no regression after stopping OCPs → resect
  - Ruptured → IR embolization, recover, then resect in elective setting

Positive sulfur colloid uptake = functioning Kupffer cells → FNH
Negative sulfur colloid uptake = absent Kupffer cells, from hepatocytes → adenoma

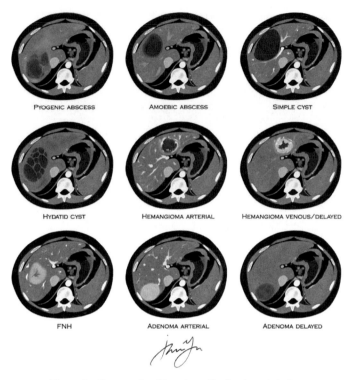

Figure 4 – Cross sectional imaging of benign hepatic lesions

- ○ What are the features of hepatocellular carcinoma (HCC)?
  - • Risk factors (causes of liver inflammation)
    - • HBV, HCV, cirrhosis of any cause, inherited errors of metabolism (hemochromatosis, alpha 1 antitrypsin deficiency), aflatoxin
  - • CT scan: hypervascular lesions; hyperintense during arterial phase; hypodense during the delayed phase
    - • Characteristic lesion on imaging + elevated AFP = no biopsy needed
  - • Is there a role for PET/CT?
    - • No role in HCC
  - • What is the most common site of metastasis?

- Lung
- What is the management?
  - Resection indicated for cure if solitary mass without major vascular invasion and adequate liver function (i.e. low grade with normal function or Childs A without portal hypertension)
    - Resection is possible but controversial for limited major vascular invasion or multifocal disease that is resectable
  - How much FLR (future liver remnant) is needed?
    - No cirrhosis → 25%
    - Childs A → 30-40%
    - What if less than above but otherwise resectable disease?
      - Consider preop portal vein embolization of diseased side
  - No cirrhosis or Childs A and early stage → resection
  - Moderate to severe cirrhosis and early stage → Transplant
    - Must meet Milan criteria:
      - One lesion < 5 cm
      - 3 or fewer lesions all less than 3 cm and no gross vascular or extrahepatic spread

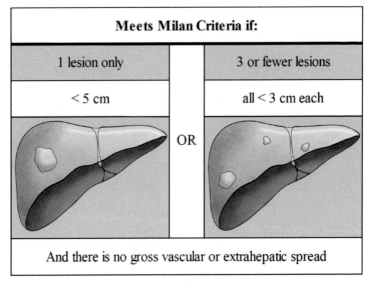

Meets Milan Criteria if:		
1 lesion only		3 or fewer lesions
< 5 cm	OR	all < 3 cm each
And there is no gross vascular or extrahepatic spread		

Figure 5 – Milan criteria

- o Usually perform neoadjuvant chemotherapy prior to transplant
- Locoregional therapies should be considered in patients who are not candidates for surgical curative treatments, or as a bridge to curative therapy
  - o Ablation (radiofrequency, cryoablation, microwave) = best for small lesions < 5 cm
  - o Arterially directed therapies – transarterial chemoembolization (TACE)
    - Consider for unresectable tumors > 5 cm
  - o External beam radiation therapy
    - Also an option for unresectable disease
    - Good for lesions not amenable to ablation or TACE due to tumor location
- o What are the features of cholangiocarcinoma?
  - Classified as intrahepatic or extrahepatic disease
  - Risk factors (inflammation of bile ducts): primary sclerosing cholangitis, bile duct stones, choledochal cysts, liver fluke infections, HBV, HCV

- What is the management of intrahepatic cholangiocarcinoma?

  - Preop biopsy is not necessary if radiographically and clinically suggested malignancy

  - Diagnostic laparoscopy to rule out disseminated disease recommended

    o Lymph node metastasis past porta hepatis and distant metastases contraindicate resection

    o Multifocal liver disease is generally not amenable to resection

> Unlike hepatocellular carcinoma, transplantation is NOT an option for multifocal cholangiocarcinoma.

  - Hepatic resection with negative margin is goal (formal anatomic resection, wedge resection, or segmental resection)

- What is the management of extrahepatic cholangiocarcinoma?

  - Basic principle is complete resection with negative margins and regional lymphadenectomy

  - Location is hilar, how do you resect?

    o In order to be resectable, contralateral hemi-liver must have intact arterial/portal flow and biliary drainage uninvolved with tumor

    o Reconstruction generally with Roux-en-Y hepaticojejunostomy

  - Location is distal, how do you resect?

    o Pancreaticoduodenectomy (Whipple)

o What are the features of gallbladder carcinoma?

- Risk factors: chronic inflammation, porcelain gallbladder (much lower risk than previously thought), polyps > 1 cm, typhoid infection, primary sclerosing cholangitis, IBD

- Many discovered incidentally at time of cholecystectomy for symptomatic gallbladder disease

- Surgical management

  - T1a tumors (invades lamina propria) →
    cholecystectomy alone

  - T1b and greater (invades muscle layer) →
    cholecystectomy with limited hepatic resection
    (typically segments IVb and V) and portal
    lymphadenectomy

    o More extensive resection may be required for
      more advanced disease in order to obtain negative
      margins

Quick Hits

- Patient with colorectal cancer and isolated liver metastasis
  receives neoadjuvant FOLFOX therapy, restaging shows
  complete radiologic response. Next step?
  o Still perform hepatic resection as complete pathologic
    response is rare

> Same principle as rectal cancer that has clinically resolved
> after neoadjuvant

- Patient with asymptomatic cholelithiasis and a 5 mm
  gallbladder polyp. Next step?
  o Cholecystectomy

  o Risk of malignant transformation within gallbladder polyps
    has been linked to concurrent cholelithiasis → surgery
    recommended regardless of polyp size if concurrent stones

- Highest negative predictive value test for choledocholithiasis?
  o GGT (beta-glutamyl transpeptidase) → normal GGT has
    97% NPV

- How do you manage choledocholithiasis in patient with prior
  Roux-en-Y gastric bypass?
  o Transgastric ERCP or advanced double-balloon endoscopy

- What is the significance of HCC found in young patient without cirrhosis?
  - Fibrolamellar variant
  - Better prognosis, recurrence is common
  - Marker?
    - Neurotensin

- Incidental finding of adenocarcinoma invading lamina propria layer of gallbladder following cholecystectomy. Next step?
  - No further treatment → cholecystectomy alone is enough

- Incidental finding of adenocarcinoma following cholecystectomy. Next step?
  - Stage
  - Go back to OR for resection of segments IVb and V and portal lymphadenectomy
  - Do you need to excise port sites?
    - No benefit

- What is the significance of isolated gastric varices?
  - Most commonly caused by splenic vein thrombosis secondary to pancreatitis
  - Treatment = splenectomy

- Patient 4 weeks after hospitalization for car accident with liver laceration that was managed nonoperatively presents with upper GI bleed. Management?
  - First step = EGD → you see blood coming from the duodenal papilla
  - What is this?
    - Hemobilia from hepatic artery-biliary duct fistula
    - Treatment = angioembolization

- What segments do you take in a right liver resection?
  - 5-8
  - Left?

- 2-4 +/- caudate (1)
  - Left lateral segmentectomy?
    - 2-3
  - Extended right?
    - 5-8 + 4
  - Extended left?
    - 2-4 + 5 and 8

08 ADRENAL

High Yield Anatomy

Vascular supply
- Superior: phrenic artery
- Middle: aorta
- Inferior: renal artery

Left vein drains into left renal vein, right vein drains into the IVC
Adrenal Cortex (Mesoderm) +Medulla (Ectoderm)
Neuroendocrine in origin chromaffin cells
- Zona Glomerulosa: "Salt" – regulates aldosterone
- Zona Fasicularis: "Sugar"- glucocorticoids
- Zona Reticularis: "Sex"- androgens/estrogen

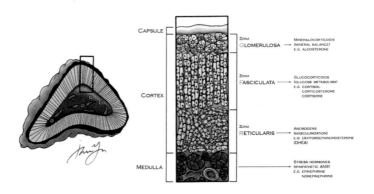

Incidentaloma:
- 1-2% found incidentally on imaging
- Concerning features of >4-6 cm, >10 HU, enlarging, and functioning
- Always look for functioning tumors before biopsy
- Send urine urine metanephrines/VMA/catecholamines, urinary hydroxycorticosteroids, serum K with plasma renin and aldosterone levels

Congenital Adrenal Hyperplasia

- 21 and 11 beta hydroxylase are crucial to convert cholesterol to aldosterone, cortisol, and testosterone
- 21 hydroxylase deficiency: increased testosterone and decreased aldosterone
- 11 hydroxylase deficiency: increased testosterone and increased aldosterone
- 17 hydroxylase deficiency: decreased testosterone and increased aldosterone

Enzyme (↓ = ↑)	Aldosterone (first number) Hypertension, hypokalemia	Testosterone (second number) Virilization
21	−	↑
17	↑	−
11	↑	↑

Hyperalderosteronism: Conn's syndrome

- Hypertension because of sodium preservation and K wasting
- Primary: renin low, Secondary: renin high
- Plasma aldosterone: renin >25
- Bilateral idiopathic adrenal hyperplasia is MC reason in 60-65% (manage medically)
- Dx: with salt load suppression test, urine aldosterone will remain elevated
- Localize on CT, MRI, NP-59 scintigraphy or Adrenal venous sampling
- Tx: spironolactones, CCB like nifedipine and K replacement
- Surgery: adrenalectomy
- If bilateral, will need fludrocortisone postoperatively

Hypocortisolism (Addison's disease)

- Decreased cortisol and aldosterone with high ACTH
- Dx: cosyntropin testing- cortisol remains low
- Acute Adrenal insufficiency: refractory hypotension, fevers, lethargy, pain, N/V

- Tx: Dexamethasone, fluids
- Chronic: Give corticosteroids

Hypercortisolism Cushing's syndrome

- Most commonly exogenous
- Measure 24-hour cortisol or urinary cortisol and late-night cortisol
- ACTH low—look for adrenal adenoma
- Adrenalectomy when dx on CT scan
- ACTH high—look for pituitary tumors (Cushing's DISEASE) or ectopic producer like small cell lung cancer
- Cushing's disease: #1 cause, Brain MRI followed by transsphenoidal approach resection
- Ectopic ACTH: #2 cause, CT CAP, resection

Adrenocortical Carcinoma

- Typically present at advanced stages, rare malignancy
- Very aggressive, patients present with Cushing syndrome, virilization and HTN
- Radical adrenalectomy with debulking, mitotane for adjuvant/ recurrent disease

Pheochromocytoma

- Rule of 10: 10% are malignant, bilateral, in children, familial, and extra-adrenal
- Only adrenal pheochromocytomas will produce epinephrine because of PNMT enzyme
- Can be seen on MIBG (when imaging does not show mass)
- Preoperative prep included volume replacement, alpha blockade with phenoxybenzamine or prazosin, followed by beta blockade
- Tx: adrenalectomy (ligate adrenal veins first to avoid spillage)
- Additional sites are paragangliomas; MC is organ of Zuckerkandl

Quick Hits

- Clonidine suppression test for patients with suspected pheochromocytoma but normotensive
- MC reason for Cushing Syndrome – Exogenous steroids
- MC reason for Addison Disease (adrenal insufficiency) – Autoimmune (1st world) or Tuberculosis (3rd world)

09 PANCREAS

Acute Pancreatitis

- Most common causes = ETOH, Gallstones

- Gallstone pancreatitis: Clear the duct (ERCP vs IOC) →
  cholecystectomy during same admission

	<4 weeks	**>4 weeks**
Non-necrotizing	Acute peri-pancreatic fluid collection	Pseudocyst
Necrotizing	Acute necrotic collection	Walled off necrosis (you WON an operation)

Table 1 - Revised Atlanta Classification for post pancreatitis fluid collections

- Necrotizing pancreatitis
  - Antibiotics?
    - No for pancreatitis
    - No for necrotizing pancreatitis
    - Yes, for necrotizing pancreatitis with signs of infection
      - Clinical signs: fever, elevated WBC
      - CT guided FNA with organisms
      - Imipenem is antibiotic of choice
  - Step-up approach — Answer for infected pancreatic necrosis used to be immediate OR for open debridement — 2010 JAMA article showed improved outcomes with delayed OR with "step-up" approach

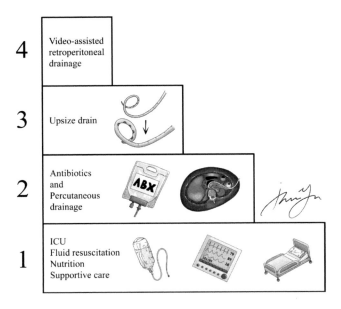

Figure 1: Step-Up Approach for Infected Pancreatic Necrosis

Chronic Pancreatitis

- Secondary to longstanding ETOH abuse, biliary tract disease, autoimmune, or idiopathic

- What are the symptoms of chronic pancreatitis?
  - ○ Persistent abdominal pain, weight loss, pancreatic insufficiency (malabsorption, steatorrhea, diabetes) with hx of one or more bouts of pancreatitis

- What is the preferred imaging and findings?
  - ○ CT can confirm diagnosis - demonstrates fibrosis, atrophy, and calcification of the gland

- Chronic pancreatitis increases risk of pancreatic cancer

- Non-operative management — pain control, nutritional management, abstaining from ETOH, pancreatic enzyme replacement

- Two main categories of operations for chronic pancreatitis: Decompress obstructed ductal system and resection of diseased tissue (Or combination of both) — several variations and very complex topic but main operations for the ABSITE are:

  o Puestow Procedure — Longitudinal pancreaticojejunostomy

  o Beger Procedure — Resection of pancreatic head up to wall of duodenum with either end to end or side to side pancreaticojejunostomy (Duodenum preserving pancreatic head resection)

  o Frey Procedure — Lateral longitudinal pancreaticojejunostomy with an excavation of the pancreatic head (Core out head of pancreas but avoid pancreatic transection required of Beger procedure)

- Operative intervention depends on particular morphology of disease

  o For dilated pancreatic duct (6mm or greater) would go with Peustow, so long as pancreatic head is normal

  o If pancreatic head dominant disease with or without duct dilation → Frey procedure

  o If distal pancreatic duct stricture with side branch changes and normal pancreatic head → distal pancreatectomy

  o Minimal change pancreatitis → Resection and/or drainage will not help → denervation operation (bilateral thoracoscopic splanchnicectomy)

Pseudocyst

- More common with chronic pancreatitis, however, can occur after acute pancreatitis

- Most will resolve spontaneously → manage expectantly for at least 6 weeks (ideally 3mo). Most will resolve in this time period, wait time also allows wall to mature. Consider intervention if >6cm or symptomatic.

- Often associated with pancreatic duct abnormality → Need ERCP or MRCP prior to intervention

- o Available approaches include transpapillary endoscopic stenting, endoscopic transluminal drainage, open cystgastrostomy, laparoscopic cystgastrostomy
- o How I would answer: If given a patient with persistent abdominal pain following pancreatitis and contained fluid collection on CT → Image ductal system FIRST (ERCP or MRCP), then if it's been at least 6 weeks open or lap cystgastrostomy.

Cystic Neoplasms of the Pancreas

- Many found incidentally on abdominal CTs done for other reasons → MRCP will provide better characterization and duct anatomy.
  - o EUS is helpful as well and allows for aspiration for cyst fluid analysis (CEA and Amylase)

- Management based on cyst characteristics and patient symptoms
  - o CEA >192 c/w mucinous cyst
  - o High amylase indicates ductal communication (pseudocyst or IPMN)

- Serous cystadenoma
  - o Predominantly benign
  - o Well circumscribed with characteristic central stellate scar on imaging
  - o Low CEA
  - o Resect only if symptomatic or growing on serial imaging

- Mucinous cystic neoplams (MCN)
  - o One of two mucinous lesions of the pancreas (along with IPMN)
  - o Have malignant potential
  - o Elevated CEA on FNA
  - o Radiographically: thick walled, single cyst with internal septations
  - o All MCNs should be resected in fit patients

- Intraductal Papillary Mucinous Neoplasm (IPMN)
  - Classification: Main Duct IPMN and Branch Duct IPMN (Mixed type managed like MD)
  - Main Duct IPMN — higher risk of malignancy than BD-IPMN
    - Endoscopic visualization of mucin secreting from a patulous "fish mouth" papilla is pathognomonic for MD IPMN
    - Surgical resection is recommended for all main duct and mixed type IPMNs
  - Branch Duct IPMN — lower risk of malignancy than MD-IPMN
    - Management based on Fukuoka guidelines
    - Decision to resect based on fitness of patient for surgery, risk tolerance of patient, and individual cyst characteristics
      - Consider resection for:
        - "Worrisome Features" — cyst size >3cm, thickened cyst wall, nonenhancing mural nodules, lyphadenopathy, MPD >10mm, abrupt change in MPD size with distal atrophy
        - EUS with mural nodules, main duct involvement, or suspicious cytology
        - Young patient with cyst >2cm owing to cumulative risk of malignancy
- Age can indicate likely lesion
  - Daughter → solid pseudopapillary
  - Mother → mucinous
  - Grandmother → serous

Neuroendocrine Tumors of the Pancreas (PNETs)

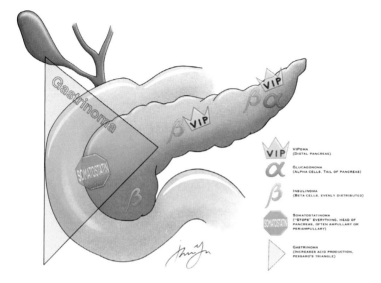

Figure 2: PNET Distribution

- Comprise 1-2% of pancreatic tumors

- Frequently non-functional, but can also elaborate a number of bioactive peptides (gastrin, glucagon, somatostatin, insulin, VIP)

- If functional, clinical presentation is characteristic of hormone elaborated

- Nonfunctional pancreatic neuroendocrine tumor
  - Majority (60-90%) of nonfunctional PNETs are <u>malignant</u>
  - Most discovered late due to asymptomatic nature. Can be discovered incidentally or 2/2 symptoms from mass effect – Generally large at time of discovery with high metastasis rate
  - MC in head of pancreas
    - Tumors <u>IN</u> the head of the pancreas: insul<u>IN</u>oma, gastr<u>IN</u>oma, somatostat<u>IN</u>oma
  - Patients with locoregional disease should undergo resection

- Insulinoma
  - Most common functional PNET
  - Insulin secreted by beta-cells
  - Most are <u>benign</u> (90%)
  - Located throughout pancreas
  - Associated with "<u>Whipple Triad</u>"
    - Fasting hypoglycemia
    - Neuroglycopenic symptoms (confusion, combativeness, seizures, visual changes, loss of consciousness)
    - Relief of symptoms with administration of glucose
  - Biochemical diagnosis and confirmation tests – If meet the below criteria, localization studies should be done
    - Symptoms with plasma glucose <55mg/dL
    - Insulin >18pmol/L
    - C-peptide ≥ 0.6 ng/mL
    - Proinsulin ≥ 5 pg/mL
    - Beta-hydroxybutyrate ≤ 2.7mmol/L
    - An increase in plasma glucose of at least 25 mg/dL after administration of glucagon
  - Localization studies
    - 1 – Triphasic CT or MRI
    - 2 – Endoscopic US
    - 3 – If above unable to localize → Selective intra-arterial calcium injection with hepatic venous sampling for insulin
    - Somatostatin scintigraphy is NOT effective
  - Treatment
    - Depends on location, suspicion for malignancy, and presence of other tumors
      - Solitary, benign appearing tumors can be treated with enucleation
      - Distal tumors may be treated with distal spleen preserving pancreatectomy
      - Suspicion for malignancy requires formal resection

- Gastrinoma
  - Gastrin stimulates acid secretion from parietal cells
  - <u>Mostly malignant</u> (60-90%)
  - 2/3rd are located in <u>Gastrinoma Triangle</u>, a triangle formed by:
    - Junction of the cystic duct and CBD
    - Junction of the 2nd and 3rd portions of the duodenum
    - Junction of the neck and body of the pancreas
  - Associated with classic triad (abdominal pain, diarrhea, weight loss) in the presence of PUD
  - Diagnostic and confirmatory tests
    - Elevated fasting serum gastrin level – must be with a low gastric pH or high basal acid output (as use of PPI or H2 blockers will raise gastrin levels)
    - Fasting gastrin level >1000 pg/mL is diagnostic
      - Elevated levels <1000 pg/mL → secretin stimulation test
        - Gastrinoma will have a paradoxical effect from secretin (Increase >200 pg/mL with administration of secretin is diagnostic)
      - Localization studies
        - 1. Triphasic CT or MRI
        - 2. Somatostatin receptor scintigraphy (SRS)
        - 3. EUS
        - 4. Possible selective intra-arterial calcium injection with hepatic venous sampling for gastrin (institution specific)
        - Unable to localize → Exploration with the following maneuvers
          - Intraoperative U/S
          - Transduodenal palpation
          - Intraoperative upper endoscopy with transduodenal illumination
          - Duodenotomy with palpation

- o Treatment
  - Tumor in duodenal mucosa → enucleation and periduodenal lymph node dissection
  - Noninvasive tumors 5cm or smaller in head of pancreas → enucleation with periduodenal lymph node dissection
  - Tumors >5cm or invasive in head of pancreas → Whipple
  - Tumor in body and tail → distal pancreatectomy

- Glucagonoma
  - o Glucagon secreted from alpha islet cells and acts on hepatocytes and adipose tissue to increase gluconeogenesis and glycogenolysis
  - o <u>Mostly malignant</u> (90%)
  - o MC location is tail of pancreas
  - o Associated with <u>4 D's – dermatitis, diabetes, depression, and DVT</u>
    - DVT 2/2 a factor X-like antigen secreted by tumor
  - o Characteristic skin rash = necrolytic migratory erythema
  - o Diagnostic and confirmatory tests
    - Glucose intolerance + fasting glucagon levels between 1,000-5,000 pg/mL
  - o Localization studies
    - Triphasic CT or MRI
    - Somatostatin receptor Scintigraphy
    - EUS
    - Selective visceral angiography
  - o Treatment
    - Resection with regional lymphadenectomy (no enucleation due to high malignant potential
      - Usually distal pancreatectomy

- What else is needed?
  - ○ Cholecystectomy (d/t possible need for prolonged somatostatin therapy)
- Somatostatinoma
  - ○ Somatostatin has a broad spectrum of inhibitory activity in the GI tract
  - ○ Mostly malignant
  - ○ MC location is head of pancreas (duodenal location also common)
  - ○ Associated with cholecystitis, DM, malabsorption, steatorrhea
  - ○ Localization studies
    - Triphasic CT or MRI
    - Somatostatin receptor scintigraphy
    - EUS
    - Selective arteriography
  - ○ Treatment
    - Resection with regional lymphadenectomy (No enucleation due to high malignant potential)
    - AND…?
      - Cholecystectomy
- VIPoma
  - ○ VIP is neuropeptide that stimulates secretion of fluids and electrolytes into lumen, also inhibits gastric acid secretion
  - ○ Mostly malignant
  - ○ MC location is body or tail of pancreas (extra-pancreatic locations also possible: adrenal, retroperitoneum, mediastinum)
  - ○ Associated with WDHA syndrome (watery diarrhea, hypokalemia, achlorhydria)
  - ○ Diagnostic tests
    - Elevated fasting VIP levels when diarrhea is present

○ Localization studies

  • Triphasic CT of MRI

  • Somatostatin receptor scintigraphy

  • EUS

  • Selective arteriography

○ Treatment

  • Resection with regional lymphadenectomy (no enucleation due to high malignant potential

  • AND???

    • Cholecystectomy (d/t possibly need for prolonged somatostatin therapy)

Most common?	Answer
Pancreatic tumor	Non-functional PNETs
Functional PNET	Insulinoma
Tumor associated with MEN1	PNETs (functional and non-functional)

Table 21: High-Yield PNET

Pancreatic Adenocarcinoma

• Risk factors: cigarette smoking, heavy ETOH use, chronic pancreatitis, increased BMI, longstanding DM

• Imaging
  ○ Pancreatic protocol CT

  ○ EUS can be complimentary to CT in patients with questionable involvement of lymph nodes or blood vessels

  ○ PET/CT used selectively if suspicion for metastasis

• Role of staging laparoscopy? – Controversial. Used routinely by some, selectively by others only in patients at high risk for disseminated disease (borderline resectable, high CA 19-9, large primary tumor, large regional nodes, highly symptomatic)

• Biopsy?
  ○ Pathologic diagnosis NOT required prior to resection

  ○ Needed prior to neoadjuvant therapy or if unresectable, prior to definitive chemotherapy

- Role of preoperative biliary drainage?
  - o No effect on survival; associated with increased wound infections rates
  - o For resectable disease and not undergoing neoadjuvant therapy → Consider only if significant pruritis, cholangitis, coagulopathic.
  - o For patients undergoing neoadjuvant therapy → drain if jaundiced
  - o What kind of stent?
    - Self-expanding metal stents are preferred because they are easy to place without dilation, have longer patency than plastic stents, and do not interfere with resection

- Resectability
  - o Resectable
    - No arterial tumor contact
    - <180-degree contact with SMV or PV without vein contour irregularity
  - o Borderline Resectable
    - Tumor contact with SMA or celiac <180 degrees
    - Tumor contact with common hepatic only (no celiac or proper hepatic involvement) allowing for resection and reconstruction
    - Involvement of SMV or PV that is amenable to resection and reconstruction
    - Tumor contact with IVC
  - o Unresectable
    - Distant metastasis
    - >180-degree contact with SMA or celiac
    - Unreconstructable involvement of SMV or PV

- Treatment
  - o Primary Surgery

- Distal tumors present late and are usually too advanced at time of diagnosis for resection → Distal pancreatectomy and splenectomy if resectable

- Head of pancreas tumor → pancreaticoduodenectomy (Whipple procedure)

- If found to be unresectable at time of operation → consider palliative biliary bypass, gastrojejunostomy, and/or celiac plexus neurolysis depending on individual tumor characteristics and patient symptoms

- In absence of frank venous occlusion PV or SMV resection and reconstruction may be performed in order to obtain R0 resection

  ○ Perioperative therapy

- Recurrence rates are high, even with R0 resection → Everyone gets adjuvant therapy

  - FOLFIRINOX (FOLinic acid, Fluorouricil, IRINotecan, OXaliplatin)

- Neoadjuvant chemoradiation should be considered for those with borderline resectable disease (requires EUS with FNA for pathologic confirmation first)

Quick Hits

- Patient with history of multiple episodes of pancreatitis now presents with hematemesis. Diagnosis and management?
  ○ Gastric varices from splenic vein thrombosis

  ○ Treatment = Splenectomy

- Patient with multiple branch duct IPMNs on imaging. There are multiple small benign appearing cysts throughout proximal pancreatic body with larger dominant one more distally with worrisome features. Management?
  ○ Resect distal lesion, okay to leave smaller benign ones behind but will need surveillance

- 48-year-old patient incidentally diagnosed with 2cm branch chain IPMN on abdominal CT. Microcytic anemia noted on laboratory w/u. What else does he/she need as part of work up?
  ○ Colonoscopy — IPMN patients have higher incidence of

extra-pancreatic malignancies (MC - Colon adenocarcinoma)

- Syndromes associated with PNETs?
  - o MEN I
    - Usually multiple PNETs – can be functional or non-functional

- MC pancreatic tumor?
  - o Nonfunctional

- MC functional tumor?
  - o Gastrinoma

- Patient presents with episodes of fasting hypoglycemia and dizziness that resolves with glucose administration. C-peptide is checked and is low. Diagnosis?
  - o Exogenous (factitious) insulin administration

- Medical management of functional neuroendocrine tumors of pancreas?
  - o Octreotide; except for…Insulinoma

- Somatic mutations associated with pancreatic adenocarcinoma?
  - o KRAS, TP53, CDKN2A, SMAD4

- Biomarkers associated with pancreatic adenocarcinoma?
  - o Many, but CA 19-9 is best validated and most clinically useful

- During pancreaticoduodenectomy for pancreatic adenocarcinoma, a clinically positive lymph node is encountered outside the field of resection. Should you:
  - o A. Leave it alone
  - o B. Perform regional lymphadenectomy
  - o C. Sample the node but not perform complete regional lymphadenectomy
    - Answer = C. Nodal metastasis are a marker of systemic disease and removal is unlikely to alter overall survival. Outside of a clinical trial a regional lymphadenectomy should not be performed during Whipple procedure.

10 COLORECTAL

High Yield Anatomy

- What are the dimensions of the colon?
  - ○ Approximately 5- 6 feet in length, with the rectum encompassing approximately 15 cm
  - ○ Normal caliber is 3-8 cm, cecal diameter > 9 cm is abnormal

- Which portions of the colon are retroperitoneal?
  - ○ Ascending
  - ○ Descending

- What is the blood supply to the colon?
  - ○ Superior mesenteric artery
    - Terminal branch = ileocolic artery → TI, cecum
    - Right and middle colic arteries → ascending and proximal 2/3rd of the transverse colon
  - ○ Inferior mesenteric artery
    - Left colic → distal 1/3rd of the transverse colon and descending
    - Sigmoid branches → sigmoid colon
    - Superior rectal artery → proximal rectum
  - ○ Collaterals
    - Marginal artery → along the colon wall connecting the SMA and IMA
    - The Arc of Riolan (meandering mesenteric artery) → smaller connection between the SMA and IMA

- What are the "watershed" areas of the colon:
  - ○ Splenic flexure – SMA/IMA connection (Griffith's point)
  - ○ Rectal/sigmoid – superior/middle rectal artery connection (Sudeck's point)

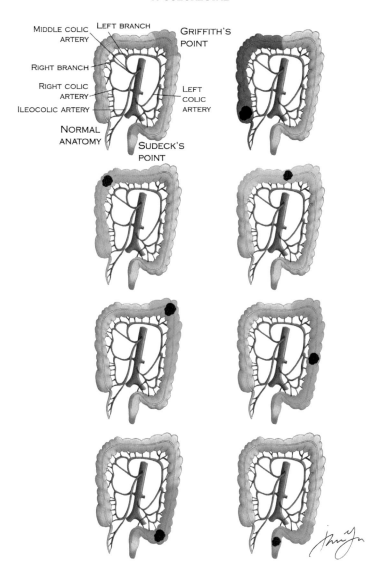

Figure 1 – Vascular anatomy of the colon with tumor resection margins

- What is the blood supply to the rectum?
  - Superior rectal (hemorrhoidal) artery - branch of IMA
  - Middle rectal (hemorrhoidal) artery - branch of internal iliac (hypogastric) artery

o Inferior rectal (hemorrhoidal) artery- branch of internal pudendal → from internal iliac

 Remember to check groin lymph nodes for low rectal cancers.

- What is the venous drainage of the rectum?
  o Superior rectal vein → IMV → portal circulation
  o Middle and Inferior rectal veins → internal iliac vein → systemic circulation

- What are the proximal and distal extents of the rectum?
  o Proximal extent starts where the taeniae splay
  o Distal extent is the anal canal (15 cm from anal verge)

- What defines the anal canal?
  o Begins at puborectalis sling (anorectal ring) → ends at anal verge = squamous mucosa blending with the perianal skin

- What defines the anal margin?
  o Extends 5 cm radially from squamous mucocutaneous junction

PART ONE

Anal Fissure

o Where do anal fissures present?
  - 90% located within posterior midline
  - Females can have anterior fissures in 25% of cases

o What is the first line treatment?
  - Non-operative management
    - Psyllium or other bulking agent, sitz baths +/- topical anesthetic
    - Topical nitrates → side effects = headaches
    - Topical calcium channel blockers have similar efficacy to nitrates without the side effects

- Botulinum toxin has modest healing rates for those who fail topical therapy

> Incontinence with botulinum injection is a contraindication for LIS.

o What are the surgical options?
- Lateral internal sphincterotomy
  - LIS has superior efficacy to nonoperative treatments, but has a small risk of fecal incontinence
  - Contraindications: women of childbearing age, prior obstetrical injuries, IBD, or history of sphincter dysfunction/incontinence
- Anocutaneous flap
  - Has inferior healing rates to LIS but lower incidence of fecal seepage/incontinence
  - Can be performed in addition to LIS or botulinum injection

Anorectal Abscess/Fistula-in-Ano

o Anorectal Abscess
- Where do anorectal abscesses occur?
  - Defined by the anatomic space they occupy
    - Intersphincteric- between the internal and external sphincter muscles
    - Ischiorectal (ischioanal)- lateral to the rectal wall in the space next to the ischial tubercle
    - Perirectal/Perianal – right around the anus
    - Supralevator – above the levator muscle
    - Submucosal – under the mucosa in the anal canal
    - Deep postanal space
      - Bilaterally ends in the ischiorectal fossa
      - "Floor" is the anococcygeal ligament
      - "Ceiling" is the levator muscle

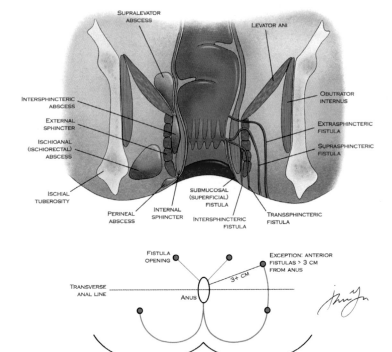

Figure 2 – Anorectal anatomy

- What is the primary treatment?
  - Drainage
    - Superficial perianal and ischiorectal – external incision and drainage
    - Deeper intersphincteric and supralevator – internal transanal drainage
  - Who needs antibiotics after drainage?
    - If there is cellulitis, systemic signs of infection, or underlying immunosuppression
  - What is the risk of developing fistula in ano?
    - One-third of patients with anal abscess will develop FIA

o Fistula in Ano (FIA)
- How are anal fistulae defined?
  - Relationship to sphincter muscles
    - Intersphincteric – most common type and runs between the internal and external sphincter muscles
    - Transsphincteric – runs across both the internal and external sphincter muscles
      - Can also be categorized as high (>1/3rd of the muscle complex) or low (< 1/3rd of the muscle complex)
    - Suprasphincteric – runs between the muscles and up and over the external sphincter
    - Extrasphincteric – runs over and above (outside) of the sphincter complex
    - Submucosal
- What are the general principles of management?
  - If superficial, simple fistula with minimal or no sphincter involvement discovered at the time of I&D for abscess → okay to perform fistulotomy at time of drainage
  - If involves more than 25% of sphincters → drain abscess and place seton
    - Seton induces fibrosis of tract
    - Goal is to convert high fistula to low fistula and prepare tract for later procedures
  - LIFT = Ligation of Intersphincteric Fistula Tract
    - Good option for fistulas not amenable to simple fistulotomy
  - Anorectal advancement flap +/- LIFT
    - Always done after seton placement

 Avoid selecting fistula plug or fibrin glue as the answer.

Hemorrhoids

o What are hemorrhoids?
- Vascular cushions or sinusoids in the anal canal that help with gross continence

o Where is the division between internal and external hemorrhoids?
- Dentate/pectinate line
- Innervation is somatic below the dentate line and autonomic above (i.e. external hemorrhoids are painful)

o What are the common symptoms of hemorrhoidal disease?
- Bleeding, swelling, thrombosis
- Internal hemorrhoids predominately prolapse and bleed
- External hemorrhoids predominately present with pain after clotting

o What is the classification of internal hemorrhoids?
- I – internal only
- II – prolapse and spontaneously reduce
- III – prolapse and manually are reducible
- IV – prolapse and are not reducible

o How do you manage hemorrhoidal disease?
- Bowel hygiene: no prolonged sitting or straining at the toilet, fiber (25-35g/day), and plenty of fluid
- Internal hemorrhoids can be banded
  - Risks- pain, bleeding, ulcer, and small risk of Fournier's gangrene
- Symptomatic/thrombosed external hemorrhoid can be excised

 Never choose banding or incision and drainage for external hemorrhoids.

Diverticulitis

o What is the Hinchey classification?

Stage	Findings	Diagram	Treatment
I	Pericolonic abscess < 4 cm		Antibiotics
II	Pelvic or inter-loop abscess, or abscess > 4 cm		Antibiotics + drain placement
III	Purulent peritonitis		Antibiotics + sigmoid colectomy
IV	Feculent peritonitis		Antibiotics + sigmoid colectomy

Table 1 – Hinchey classification of diverticulitis

o What constitutes complicated disease?
  - Perforation, abscess, fistula, obstruction, stricture
  - Phlegmon (contained area of inflammation) or extra-luminal gas alone does NOT constitute complicated disease

o What is the management of a clinically stable, reliable patient with uncomplicated disease who can tolerate oral hydration?
  - Outpatient treatment with oral antibiotics to cover gram + and gram − (e.g. amoxicillin/clavulanate, levofloxacin/ metronidazole)

o What about a patient with complicated disease or who cannot tolerate oral hydration?
  - This requires admission, IV hydration, and IV antibiotics (piperacillin/tazobactam or levofloxacin/metronidazole)
  - May require operative or percutaneous intervention

o How about a patient presenting unstable and/or with diffuse peritonitis?
  • OR for urgent sigmoid colectomy
  • While there is literature to support primary anastomosis in select patients even in Hinchey III/IV disease, safest answer is Hartmann's

 Avoid selecting laparoscopic lavage. If in the OR urgently/ emergently → resect.

o What if the patient is stable with an abscess?
  • Depends on the size and somewhat controversial, but in general:
    • < 3 cm generally resolve with antibiotics
    • > 3 cm should consider percutaneous drainage
  • What if the abscess is inaccessible by IR and not resolving with medical management?
    • May be candidate for laparoscopic drain placement
  • Goal is to let acute phase resolve so patient may undergo elective, single stage colectomy at later date

o Patient with single episode of uncomplicated diverticulitis diagnosed on abdominal CT was successfully treated nonoperatively. What is the next step?
  • If no recent colonoscopy → needs colonoscopy, typically 6 weeks after resolution of episode
  • To rule out underlying ischemia, IBD, or neoplasm

o When would you recommend an elective sigmoid colectomy?
  • For uncomplicated disease:
    • Difficult question - used to be based on number of episodes and age; however, we now know that the 1st episode tends to be the worst and multiple uncomplicated episodes does not necessarily increase the risk of needing an emergent colectomy and stoma
    • Decision for elective colectomy is now highly individualized

- Consider individual risk of surgery based on co-morbidities and general health of patient
- Effect of diverticulitis episodes on lifestyle and career
- Suspicion for neoplasm?
- Chronic symptoms (smoldering disease)?
- Complicated disease
  - Elective colectomy should generally be offered to patients after recovery from a complicated episode of diverticulitis.

Clostridium Difficile Infection (CDI)

o What is clostridium difficile?
- Anaerobic, gram positive rod

o What is the medical management?
- Metronidazole (500 mg TID) and vancomycin (125 mg QID) are first line oral options
  - Previously, metronidazole was first line for mild to moderate disease and vancomycin was first line for severe disease
  - Vancomycin is now first line with fidaxomicin as the alternative
  - Vancomycin enemas are also an option
- Fidaxomicin = oral macrolide with activity against resistant strains, usually requires ID consult
  - Probably not the answer on the boards
- Patients with refractory CDI can be considered for fecal transplant if conventional methods have failed

o When is surgery required?
- Surgery reserved for severe colitis that fails to respond to medical therapy
  - Outside of obvious indications like perforation and generalized peritonitis, the decision to operate can be very difficult
  - Multisystem organ failure is an ominous sign – you've waited too long; perforation is also associated with high mortality

- Consider early operative intervention in patients requiring vasopressors or signs of impending sepsis
- What is the procedure of choice?
  - Subtotal colectomy with ileostomy

A diverting loop ileostomy with colonic lavage and antegrade vancomycin enemas is another surgical option, but not on the exam.

Colonic Volvulus

o Sigmoid volvulus
  - What is the radiographic finding on plain films?
    - Bent inner tube sign – apex points to RUQ
  - What are your next steps?
    - Contrast enhanced CT to confirm diagnosis and assess colon viability
    - If no colonic ischemia or perforation on CT → endoscopic detorsion with decompression tube left in place for 1-3 days
      - High long-term recurrence rate after initial endoscopic detorsion → consider sigmoid colectomy during index admission in appropriate patients
  - What operation do you perform if emergent indications?
    - Safest answer = open sigmoidectomy with end colostomy (Hartmann)
  - What operation do you perform in the semi-elective setting after successful detorsion?
    - Open sigmoid colectomy with anastomosis

Case scenario is usually an elderly, nursing home patient on antipsychotics with history of constipation.

o Cecal volvulus
  - What is the radiographic finding?

- Coffee bean pointing to the left upper quadrant
- How do you manage this?
  - Endoscopic reduction is NOT recommended – rarely successful with high recurrence
  - These patients need to go to OR → resect if dead bowel
- How do you decide on resection vs pexy?
  - Data is limited - resection has lower recurrence but may have higher procedure-related morbidity than pexy
  - Both are acceptable answers
  - Safest answer = resection (ileocececectomy or right hemicolectomy) with primary anastomosis

> Never choose cecostomy, endoscopic detorsion, or operative detorsion alone.

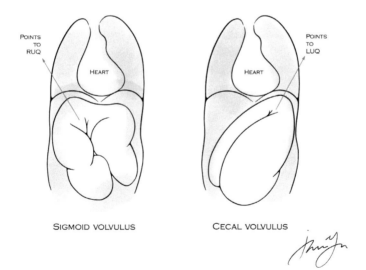

SIGMOID VOLVULUS   CECAL VOLVULUS

Figure 3 – Appearance of colonic volvulus on plain film

Acute Colonic Pseudo-Obstruction (Ogilvie's)

o What are the risk factors for Ogilvie's?
  • High dose opiates, electrolyte abnormalities, etc.

o What are the risk factors for perforation?
  • Cecum > 12 cm or duration > 6 days

o What is the initial treatment if no signs of ischemia and cecum < 12 cm?
  • Supportive care and correct underlying cause: correct electrolytes, fluid resuscitation, minimize narcotics and anticholinergic medications, treat infection, bowel rest and decompression

o What if patient is not improving with supportive care?
  • Neostigmine = anti-acetylcholinesterase, promotes colonic transit
  • What is the most common side effect?
    • Bradycardia → need to give in a monitored setting

o What if the patient is not responsive to neostigmine or neostigmine is contraindicated?
  • Endoscopic decompression

o How do you manage ischemia or perforation?
  • OR for resection (ostomy vs anastomosis +/- diversion on case by case basis)

Rectal Prolapse

o How do you diagnose rectal prolapse?
  • Full thickness intussusception of the rectal wall with visible concentric rings (important to differentiate from prolapsed hemorrhoids)

o What is the common patient presentation?
  • Higher incidence in elderly females, developmentally delayed, and psychiatric co-morbidities with multiple meds, straining and chronic diarrhea

o What are the goals of surgery?

- Eliminate prolapse through either resection or restoration of normal anatomy
- Correct associated functional abnormalities
- Avoid creation of de novo bowel dysfunction

o What is the mainstay of treatment?
  - Surgery
    - Low risk– Transabdominal rectal fixation (rectopexy)
      - Open vs laparoscopic have equivalent recurrence rates, improved morbidity with laparoscopic approach
      - Rectopexy is the key component
      - If patient has constipation → add LAR or sigmoid resection to rectopexy
    - High risk (older, multiple co-morbidities, cannot tolerate general anesthetic) – Perineal proctosigmoidectomy (Altemeier procedure)
      - Lower morbidity but higher recurrence and less durable
    - High fiber diet

Quick Hits

- What is the main nutrient of colonocytes?
  o Butyrate (short chain fatty acids)

 | Glutamine is the primary source for small bowel enterocytes.

- Patient with sigmoid volvulus on CT → on endoscopy mucosa is dusky with ulceration. Next step?
  o Abort endoscopy → OR for urgent sigmoidectomy

- Patient with anal fissure lateral or multiple fissures. What do you worry about?

    o Crohn's disease, HIV, syphilis, tuberculosis

- You take septic patient with fulminant C diff colitis to ex lap for planned total abdominal colectomy but upon opening the colon looks normal. What do you do?
  - C diff is mucosal disease → proceed with TAC and end ileostomy

- What is the management of a lower GI bleed?
  - 1st steps – Resuscitate – 2 large bore IVs, type and cross, transfuse, admit to ICU for monitoring
  - Localize the source –
    - R/o upper GI source – NG lavage
    - Colonoscopy, angiography, and/or tagged RBC scan
    - Recommendations of which to perform first vary and are institution specific – would say colonoscopy on test if it's an option
    - Most will stop spontaneously → If stops initially and then rebleeds can try 2nd attempt at localization as long as patient is stable
  - If patient unstable and/or ongoing transfusion requirement
    - Segmental colectomy if bleeding source localized by colonoscopy, angiography, or tagged RBC scan
    - TAC if unable to localize

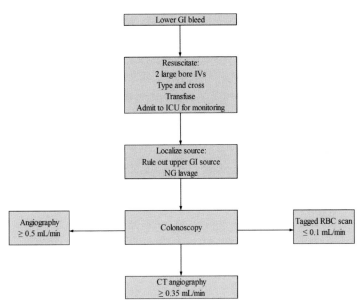

Figure 4 – **Management approach for lower GI bleed**

PART TWO

Ulcerative Colitis

o How is UC defined?

- Chronic inflammatory condition affecting rectum and extending proximally (spares anus)

- Buzzwords: mucosal disease, contiguous, characteristic crypt abscesses and pseudopolyps

o What is the management?

- Most can be managed medically with 15-30% eventually requiring surgery

- Steroids for acute flares, mesalamine maintenance, infliximab added if resistant

o What are indications for surgical intervention?

- Medical intractability (most common), malignancy, and other complications from colitis (stricture, perforation, fulminant/ toxic colitis)

- o What constitutes "medical intractability?"
- Growth failure in children
- Condition worsens while on medical therapy
- Condition is insufficiently controlled with maximal medical therapy – somewhat vague, but essentially patient can't achieve adequate quality of life
- Risk of chronic medical therapy is not tolerated (e.g. chronic steroids)
- Disabling extra-intestinal manifestations that may respond to colectomy (e.g. large joint arthropathy, erythema nodosum, episcleritis)
  - What about hepatobiliary manifestations?
    - Typically, do NOT respond to colectomy (e.g. primary sclerosing cholangitis)
- o What is the association between UC and malignancy?
  - Increased risk of malignancy associated with prolonged inflammation
  - Surveillance recommendations;
    - Patients with extensive colitis (proximal to splenic flexure)
      - Endoscopy after 8 years of disease and then every 1-2 years
      - 4 quadrant random biopsy should be performed at 10 cm intervals throughout involved segment of colon – along with directed biopsies of suspicion lesions
    - What do you do if there is malignancy or high-grade dysplasia?
      - Total proctocolectomy with or without IPAA
- o What are the surgical options?
  - If emergent (toxic colitis, perforation, etc.) → total or subtotal colectomy with end ileostomy
    - Later may perform completion proctectomy and IPAA

- Elective options
  - Total proctocolectomy with end ileostomy = curative, removes all pathologic tissue
  - Commits patient to lifelong ileostomy
- Total proctocolectomy with IPAA – MC procedure in elective setting
  - Advantage of no stoma, but may have complications related to pouch (e.g. pouchitis)
  - Must have good baseline continence prior to IPAA
  - Must be sure it's UC and not Crohn's (Distal ileum used for ileal pouch)
- TAC with ileorectal anastomosis
  - Only used in highly select cases
  - Must have uninvolved rectum (rare)
  - Rectum still at risk for ongoing disease and risk of CA → Needs annual surveillance of residual rectal cuff

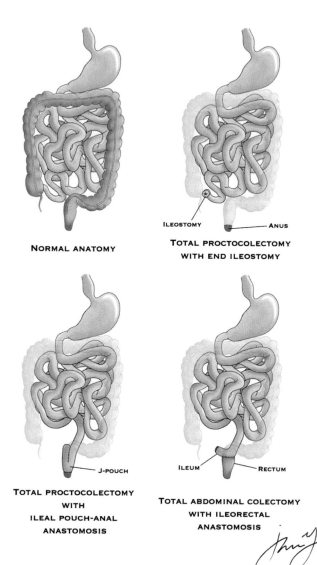

NORMAL ANATOMY

TOTAL PROCTOCOLECTOMY
WITH END ILEOSTOMY

ILEOSTOMY — ANUS

TOTAL PROCTOCOLECTOMY
WITH
ILEAL POUCH-ANAL
ANASTOMOSIS

J-POUCH

TOTAL ABDOMINAL COLECTOMY
WITH ILEORECTAL
ANASTOMOSIS

ILEUM — RECTUM

Figure 5 – Operative options for ulcerative colitis

Crohn's Disease

o How is Crohn's disease described?

- Chronic, incurable, inflammatory disorder that can affect any segment of the intestinal tract (TI most common, usually spares rectum)
- Bimodal distribution (20-30s; 50-60s)
- Buzzwords: transmural involvement, segmental, characteristic creeping fat

> UC is limited to the mucosa and affects the colon continuously.

- Phenotypes: inflammatory, fibrostenotic, penetrating (can overlap and change)
- Extraintestinal manifestations – arthritis/arthralgias, megaloblastic anemia (2/2 malabsorption of B12 in TI), uveitis, erythema nodosum

o What is the medical treatment?
  - Steroids for acute flares, 5-ASA/mesalamine for maintenance, infliximab for resistant disease

o When is surgery indicated?
  - Surgery is not curative unlike UC
  - Reserved for complications of disease – stricturing, obstruction, malignancy, perforation, fistula
  - Preserve as much small bowel as possible (often need multiple resections over course of lifetime)

o What is the management of symptomatic strictures?
  - If able to reach endoscopically – can try endoscopic dilation first
  - Otherwise – resection or stricturoplasty
    - Resection is most commonly performed – especially if isolated short segment disease
    - Stricturoplasty is useful for preserving bowel length if there is concern for existing or impending short gut
      - Type of stricturoplasty depends on length of stricture:
        - Short strictures (< 10 cm) – Heineke-Mikulicz stricturoplasty

- Longitudinal incision on stricture and close transversely
- Medium-length strictures (10-20 cm) – Finney stricturoplasty

  - Fold strictured segment on itself and make a common channel in the loop
- Long strictures (> 20 cm) – Michelassi

  - Similar to Finney – side-to-side isoperistaltic stricturoplasty
- Perform biopsies of strictured segment – Don't inadvertently leave a malignancy behind for the sake of preserving bowel length
- Malnutrition, presence of inflammation/ perforation/fistula, and suspicion for malignancy are contraindications for stricturoplasty

Colon Cancer

o What are the screening recommendations?

Risk factor	Age to start screening (yrs)	Modality	Frequency
Asymptomatic and average risk	50	Colonoscopy	Every 10 years
		Sigmoidoscopy + FOBT	Every 5 years
1° relative with colorectal CA or adenomas < 60 yrs	40 or 10 years before age of earliest diagnosed	Colonoscopy	Every 5 years
One 1° > 60 yrs or two 2° with colon cancer	40	Colonoscopy	Every 10 years
One 2° with colorectal cancer (average risk)	50	Colonoscopy	Every 10 years
FAP	10-12	Sigmoidoscopy	Yearly
Hereditary nonpolyposis colorectal CA	20-25 or 10 years before age of earliest diagnosed	Colonoscopy	Every 1-2 years

Table 2 – Colorectal cancer screening recommendations

o If patient has a personal history of adenomas what is the recommended surveillance interval?

Findings on colonoscopy	Interval to repeat
1 - 2 tubular adenomas	5 years
> 3 adenomas	3 years
Advanced adenomas (> 1 cm, high grade, dysplasia, villous)	3 years
Hyperplastic polyps (considered average risk)	10 years

Table 3 – Colonoscopy surveillance recommendations

- What if a malignant polyp was found?
  - Malignant pedunculated or sessile polyps may be managed endoscopically if the following criteria are met:
    - Polyp can be removed in 1 piece
    - Resection margins free of dysplasia or cancer
    - Lesion is well or moderately differentiated and no angiolymphatic invasion
    - Limited submucosal invasion (cancer cells 2mm or less past muscularis mucosa)
  - Malignant polyps that do not meet low-risk criteria or cannot be adequately removed via endoscopic techniques → oncologic resection

o One of the few cancers that you absolutely need to know the staging. What is the TNM staging?

Tumor Stage	Tis	Involves only lamina propria	**AJCC staging**	Stage I	T1-2 N0 M0
	T1	Invades submucosa			
	T2	Invades muscularis propria			
	T3	Invades through muscularis propria into pericolonic tissue		Stage II	T3-4 N0 M0
	T4 a	Penetrates serosa			
	b	Invades or is adherent to surrounding structures			
Nodal Stage	N1	1-3 nodes		Stage III	Any T N1-2 M0
	N2 a	4-6 nodes			
	b	7+ nodes			
M Stage	M0	No distant metastasis		Stage IV	Any T Any N M1
	M1	Distant metastasis			

Table 4 – Colon cancer staging

- Positive lymph node defined as 0.2 mm deposit of cancer cells

o What extent of proximal and distal margin is required?
  - Ideally 5-7 cm to ensure adequate lymphadenectomy

o How many nodes are needed?
  - At least 12

o What is the management of Stage IV disease?
  - Should classify as 1) resectable, 2) potentially resectable (if able to downstage with standard chemotherapy regimens), or 3) unresectable
  - Resectable
    - In medically fit patients, curative resection of hepatic and/ or pulmonary metastases can be performed
      - Sequence of chemotherapy, resection of primary tumor, and resection of metastasis varies widely by surgeon, institution, and individual patient/tumor characteristics
      - Safe answer if given resectable colon CA with hepatic metastasis: 3 months of preoperative FOLFOX → surgery → 3 months of postop FOLFOX

- Potentially resectable disease should receive preoperative FOLFOX → re-evaluate resectability based on response
- Unresectable
  - Surgery only for palliation (obstruction, bleeding, perforation)
    - If obstruction → stenting is preferable to colectomy or diversion

o Adjuvant therapy
  - Who gets adjuvant therapy?
    - In general, Stage III and above (positive nodes or M1)

> Adjuvant therapy for "high-risk" stage II disease (T4 primary, perforation/obstruction, poorly differentiated, <12 nodes harvested) is not standard of care.

- What is the regimen?
  - FOLFOX for 6 months (or 3 mo preop + 3 mo postop)
    - Folinic acid (leucovorin)
    - Fluorouracil (5-FU)
    - Oxaliplatin
- Radiation is not indicated for colon cancer

Rectal Cancer

o What is the workup for newly diagnosed rectal cancer?
  - Labs including CEA
  - Rigid proctoscopy to document level of tumor
  - CT chest/abdomen/pelvis to evaluate metastatic disease
  - Endorectal U/S (EUS) or Rectal MRI for T and N stage
    - MRI is particularly helpful in determining tumor circumferential margin (CRM)
      - CRM = total distance between tumor and mesorectal fascia
        - Very important prognostic indicator

o Who gets neoadjuvant chemoradiotherapy?

- Locally advanced tumors of mid-distal rectum (T3 or greater or any N+ disease)

- What is the regimen?

  - 5000 cGy radiotherapy delivered concurrently with 5-FU chemotherapy delivered over 5-6 weeks → surgery to follow roughly 8-12 weeks after

    - 5-FU is a radiosensitizer

o Surgical Management

- When is local excision an option?

  - Consider for T1 lesions without high-risk features

    - Well to moderately differentiated lesions, no lymphovascular or perineural invasion, < 3 cm, and < 1/3rd of circumference of bowel lumen

  - Big issue here is not able to pathologically examine regional lymph nodes

  - Patient counseling is key: up to 20% local recurrence rate for T1 lesions

    - If good surgical candidate wound lean toward resection

> Local excision can be performed for T2 lesions in poor surgical candidates but is likely not the correct answer for the exam.

- How do you manage tumors of upper 3rd of rectum?

  - Tumor specific mesorectal excision with 5 cm distal margin

- What about tumors of the mid to lower 3rd of rectum?

  - Total mesorectal excision (TME) as part of LAR or APR

  - With TME – 2 cm distal margins are ideal, 1 cm okay if very distal

    - If can't get this margin with sphincter preservation → needs APR o What is the adjuvant therapy?

- FOLFOX recommended for:

  - Stage III or greater who did not receive neoadjuvant (in other words, patient was understaged during preop w/u)

  - High-risk stage II or greater who received neoadjuvant therapy

    - In this case, we assume that pathologic high-grade stage II disease is the result of downstaging by neoadjuvant therapy

Anal Squamous Neoplasms

o How will these be described?

- Histologic variants: cloacogenic, basaloid, epidermoid, mucoepidermoid

- You need to know these because they will try to trick you by giving you a patient with an anal mass that was biopsied, and path returns as one of these variants. Recognize that you are dealing with anal SCC

  - They try to get you to do an APR when what the patient needs is primary chemoradiotherapy (Nigro).

o What HPV serotypes are associated with anal SCC?

- 16 and 18

o Who has a higher incidence of anal SCC?

- Immunosuppressed patients

o What is anal intraepithelial neoplasm (AIN)

- Precursor lesion to SCC

- Many confusing classification systems exist

- Know this:

  - AIN I, II, and III correspond to low-moderate-high grade dysplasia, respectively

  - Low grade AIN (LGAIN) = AIN I/II

  - High grade AIN (HGAIN) = AIN III

o What is the primary treatment for SCC of anal canal?

- Chemoradiotherapy (Nigro Protocol)
  - 5-FU, Mitomycin C, and 3000 cGy XRT

o What do you do with persistent or recurrent SCC of anal canal after primary CRT?
  - APR

o How do you manage SCC of the anal margin?
  - Treat like skin CA → WLE

> The anal margin extends 5 cm radially from the squamous mucocutaneous junction.

o What is the treatment of HGAIN/LGAIN?
  - Overall low rate of conversion to SCC (higher in immunosuppressed)
  - Several local treatments can be used:
    - Topical 5% imiquimod
    - Topical 5% 5-FU
    - Photodynamic therapy
    - Targeted destruction
  - Probably most important part of any of above treatments is close clinical f/u with surveillance every 4-6 months
    - Some advocate observation with surveillance alone

o Anal melanoma is treated with APR

Quick Hits

- Transverse colon cancer with local invasion of head of pancreas, no evidence of metastatic disease. How do you treat?
  o Resect en bloc: Whipple + extended hemicolectomy

- Treatment of isolated peritoneal carcinomatosis 2/2 colon CA?
  o Carcinomatosis often associated with widespread metastasis. However, if isolated → cytoreductive surgery with intraperitoneal chemotherapy

- What do you do with rectal cancer with apparent complete clinical response to neoadjuvant therapy?
  - Current imaging (CT, MRI, PET) cannot reliably predict complete clinical response → this patient still requires resection

- Patient referred for "hemorrhoid." On exam has 1 cm palpable mass of anal canal. Biopsy performed in clinic returns epidermoid carcinoma. Management?
  - Primary chemoradiotherapy (Nigro protocol)
  - This is a variant of SCC

- Patient with prior proctocolectomy and IPAA for UC presents with fever, pelvic pain, and increased frequency of stools. Flexible endoscopy shows mucosal inflammation of ileal pouch. Diagnosis?
  - Pouchitis
  - Treatment?
    - Antibiotics (ciprofloxacin/metronidazole), supportive care
      - Budesonide enemas if not responsive to antibiotics
  - Chronic pouchitis → suspect Crohn's
  - Severe refractory pouchitis may require pouch excision and ileostomy

- During laparoscopic exploration for presumed acute appendicitis, appendix appears normal, but TI inflamed. What do you do?
  - Suspect Crohn's
  - If cecum uninvolved → appendectomy to prevent future diagnostic confusion
  - If cecum inflamed → leave appendix in place
  - Either way, treat medically for acute Crohn's flare.

11 VASCULAR

Carotid/Vertebral

- What are the structures of the carotid sheath?
  - o Carotid Artery
  - o Internal Jugular Vein
  - o Vagus Nerve

- What are the segments of the vertebral artery?
  - o V1 - Origin off subclavian to foramina of C6
  - o V2 (Foraminal) - From the transverse foramen of C2-C6
  - o V3 - From C2 to Dura
  - o V4 – Intracranial

- What is the structure commonly overlies the carotid artery bifurcation?
  - o Facial vein off of IJ generally overlies the bifurcation

- What is the first branch of the external carotid artery?
  - o Superior thyroid artery

- Is the external carotid artery flow high or low resistance ?
  - o It is high resistance (flows to muscular facial muscles), so triphasic flow on doppler, brief reversal of flow

- Can the external carotid artery be ligated?
  - o External carotid can be tied off to help control excessive facial bleeding in trauma

- Internal carotid artery main blood supply to brain, first branch is the ophthalmic
  - o Low resistance as it is supplying brain tissue, so it has continuous forward flow which creates a biphasic doppler signal

Doppler of the internal carotid is biphasic with a long diastolic phase, distinctly different than the high resistance of the triphasic external carotid

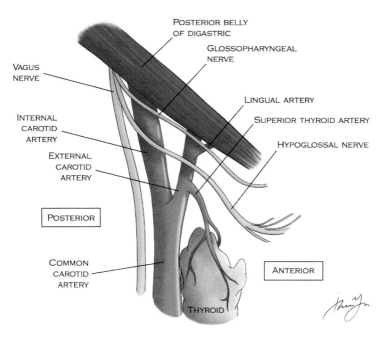

Figure 1. Carotid Bifurcation Anatomy

- Hoarseness after carotid endarterectomy?
  - Likely injury to vagus nerve
  - From clamping the carotid the vagus nerve was also clamped

- Tongue deviation to side of injury?
  - Likely hypoglossal nerve injury
  - Nerve lies just cephalad to carotid bifurcation so can easily be damaged

- Ipsilateral mouth droop after a carotid?
  - Marginal mandibular injury
  - From retraction on mandible, generally when trying to expose high lesions

- This nerve lies deep to posterior belly of digastric and if divided can cause disabling dysphagia.
  - Glossopharyngeal

- What layers of carotid are removed during an endarterectomy?
  - Intima and part of the media

- What is the typical location of carotid atherosclerosis?
  - Carotid bifurcation due to turbulence

- Indications for performing carotid endarterectomy
  - Symptomatic (stroke or TIA), 50-70% warrants surgery
  - Asymptomatic – controversial if over 80% or EDV (end diastolic velocity) > 140 cm/s (which correlates with 80% stenosis)
    - Should start with medical management aspirin and a statin

- What if patient is symptomatic but duplex shows <50% stenosis?
  - No surgery indicated
  - Optimize medical management – aspirin, Plavix and a statin

- What if patient has a stroke and imaging shows a completely occluded carotid artery?
  - Anticoagulation to prevent progression, no benefit to recanalizing

- What situations would an emergent carotid endarterectomy be indicated
  - Crescendo TIAs
    - TIA symptoms are recurring and becoming more severe or lasting longer in duration

- What is the most common non stroke cause of morbidity and mortality after CEA
  - Myocardial infarction

- When should you operate on a symptomatic carotid
  - Small stroke or TIA – within two weeks once symptoms resolve
  - Hemorrhagic stroke – 6-8 weeks

- What if patient demonstrates symptoms of stroke in PACU after carotid endarterectomy
  - Return to OR to evaluate for intimal flaps or thrombus
  - In OR start with US

- Which clinical scenarios would you consider carotid stenting over carotid endarterectomy
  - Hx of neck dissection, neck irradiation, recurrent carotid disease
  - Severe cardiac disease

> TCAR (Transcarotid Artery Revascularization) or transfemoral stenting should be considered in patients with previous neck surgery or radiation. TCAR has lowest stroke rate.

Non-Atherosclerotic Carotid Lesions

- A patient s/p blunt trauma and is found to have asymptomatic carotid dissection
  - Should be anticoagulated (either heparin or Plavix, not standardized)
  - Repeat imaging before leaving hospital

- A patient s/p blunt trauma and found to have a symptomatic dissection
  - Will likely require a covered stent

- A patient s/p blunt trauma with traumatic occlusion of carotid artery
  - If already have neurologic injury/completed stroke unlikely to get better with intervention
  - Antithrombotic therapy

- Carotid body tumors
  - All require resection
  - Consider embolization prior to surgery due to risk of bleeding

Subclavian/Thoracic Outlet

- Name the structures of the thoracic outlet anterior to posterior
  - Subclavian vein
  - Phrenic nerve
  - Anterior scalene
  - Subclavian artery
  - Middle scalene
  - First Rib

- What anatomic anomaly puts patients at risk for thoracic outlet syndrome?
  - Cervical rib

- Where is brachial plexus found in the thoracic outlet?
  - The brachial plexus is along the middle scalene, posterior to the subclavian artery

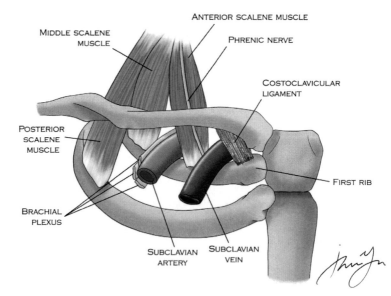

Figure 2. Thoracic Outlet Anatomy

- Which type of TOS is most common, and what are the classic symptoms?
  - Neurogenic (95%)
  - Pain, weakness, numbness and tingling in the hand, particularly in ulnar distribution
  - Symptoms worse with manipulation/elevation of arm

- Treatment of neurogenic TOS?
  - Physical therapy is go to method
  - If PT fails confirm diagnosis with scalene block or nerve conduction test
  - First rib resection and scalenectomy with neurolysis is operation of choice for refractory neurogenic TOS

- A swimmer presents with a blue swollen arm, what is this and how do you treat it?
  - Subclavian Vein Thrombosis (Paget-Schroetter), compression at costoclavicular junction
  - Treat with catheter directed thrombolysis followed by first rib resection within the same hospital stay or shortly after

- A young person with no atherosclerotic risks factors presents with ischemia of the hand
  - Common presentation for arterial TOS, though arterial TOS is very rare
  - Likely an anomalous cervical rib is compressing the subclavian artery and will lead to an aneurysm, which is an embolic risk
  - Will need first rib resection with interposition graft for the artery

Subclavian Steal Syndrome

- Where is the anatomic stenosis that results in subclavian steal?
  - Proximal subclavian narrowing
  - Results in a reversal of blood flow in vertebral, which can lead to vertebrobasilar symptoms

- o Symptoms occur when extremity is exerted and it steals blood from cerebral circulation

- How do you fix it?
  - o Endovascular recanalization and stenting or potentially carotid subclavian bypass are subclavian transposition

Dialysis Access

- How long should a temporary catheter be left in place (called Vas-Cath at many places) and why do they need to be removed?
  - o 3 weeks

  - o Infection risk

- How do long term tunneled catheters differ (Permacath)
  - o They are cuffed

  - o They are tunneled

  - o Lower risk of central infection

  - o Still higher infection rate, and high risk of central venous stenosis compared with fistula or graft

- What is preferred location for temporary dialysis access and what should be taken into account?
  - o Right IJ direct to right atrium

  - o Avoid the side where you plan to place permanent AV Fistula

  - o Will cause central venous stenosis, will lead to failure of permanent access

- What is preferred location for AV fistula creation for dialysis access?
  - o "Fistula First" Always start distal on non-dominant arm, and upper extremities before lower extremities, Start distal to not burn bridges.

  - o Reducing catheter days, improves life expectancy

  - o Focus is now moving to choosing the right access for the right person, a person with a short life expectancy, a fistula may not be the best access

- What is the most common reason for AV fistulas to malfunction over time?
  - The major cause of hemodialysis AV access failure is venous outflow problems.

- A patient reports that she is having high venous return pressures, and increased bleeding after dialysis, what is the likely problem, how do you diagnose it and what is the treatment?
  - Likely has venous outflow stenosis
  - Can be diagnosed with duplex US
  - Fistulogram with balloon angioplasty can likely correct the lesion

- What are criteria for fistula maturation, "Rule of 6s"?
  - Needs to be 6 mm in diameter
  - <6 mm deep
  - >600 mL/min in flow

- 6 weeks after a brachio-cephalic fistula creation, the fistula fails to mature, what are some likely causes of this and how can they be managed?
  - Possible inadequate inflow, rule out stricture at anastomosis, potential balloon angioplasty vs revision of anastomosis
  - Competing flow from side branches, branches need to be ligated or coiled

A bleeding fistula with pinpoint hole bleeding can be treated with a stitch and urgent fistulogram. Bleeding from an ulcer on a fistula is a surgical emergency.

Fasciotomies

- When are fasciotomies indicated? What are the symptoms?
  - In a patient with documented lower extremity compartment syndrome
  - A patient that had acute limb ischemia for > 4 hours, should be considered for prophylactic fasciotomy
  - Patients will have tight compartments, pain with passive motion of foot

- Where to make incision to access anterior and lateral compartments?
  - Make incision lateral to tibia in between the tibia and fibula (H type incision to pen both anterior and lateral compartments, incisions should be anterior and posterior to intermuscular septum.

- What nerve can you injure with the lateral incision and what deficit would you see?
  - Superficial peroneal nerve which can lead to difficulties with foot eversion.

- To access superficial posterior and deep posterior compartments?
  - Make incision two centimeters posterior/medial to tibia
  - The key to perform a complete four-compartment fasciotomy is to make sure that the posterior deep compartment has been fully decompressed. Both the superficial and the deep posterior compartments are decompressed through the medial incision.

- How do you release the deep posterior compartment?
  - Take soleus off of the tibia.

Thoracic Aorta

- In a blunt thoracic aortic injury, where is the most common site of injury?
  - Just distal to subclavian artery in the descending thoracic aorta, at the level of the ligamentum arteriosum, the aorta is tethered here

- A pseudoaneurysm develops here (partial transection)
- Treated with TEVAR

- What are the size criteria for treating descending thoracic aortic aneurysms?
  - If endovascular repair is possible if > 5.5 cm
  - Otherwise aorta should be > 6.5 cm

- What is a feared complication of thoracic aorta repairs?
  - Paraplegia (<5% for endovascular vs 20% for open)
  - Reduce this risk by placing lumbar drains and increasing the blood pressure
  - Spinal Perfusion Pressure = MAP (drive up with pressors) – ICP (lower with spinal drain)

Abdominal Aorta/Aneurysms

- Acute mesenteric ischemia has 4 types
  - Embolic
  - Thrombotic
  - Venous thrombosis
  - Non occlusive mesenteric ischemia

- Which is most common type of mesenteric ischemia and how do you diagnose and treat it
  - Embolic is most common, likely from afib or endocarditis
  - Patients will have severe abdominal pain, with no other supporting findings on exam (pain out of proportion to exam)
  - CTA is best modality to diagnose
  - Heparinize the patient and take to OR for ex lap and SMA embolectomy
  - Best to leave abdomen open and re-explore in 12-24 hours before resecting any marginally perfused bowel

- Which type is most common in a patient that has severe atherosclerotic disease burden?
  - Thrombotic disease
  - This likely occurs at ostium/takeoff of the SMA

- o Embolic disease is more distal, generally at first branch of SMA

- o Pts with thrombotic AMI, likely have had unrecognized symptoms for months – years

- o These patients will likely require a mesenteric bypass rather than embolectomy

- Which disease process embolic vs thrombotic will have proximal jejunal sparing?
  - o Embolic because it lodges just distal to first branch of SMA (3-10 cm distal to ostium)
  - o Thrombotic patients will not have any sparing of small intestine

- How do you identify the SMA to perform embolectomy?
  - o Lift transverse colon cephalad and follow to base of transverse mesocolon
  - o Just to the right of Ligament of Treitz (LOT) will be the SMA
  - o Mobilize LOT to access SMA at its origin

- What are characteristics of mesenteric venous thrombosis
  - o Sub-acute, multiple days of abdominal pain and bloody diarrhea
  - o Generally have an underlying hypercoaguable disorder
  - o CTA will demonstrate small bowel wall thickening, mesenteric edema, and thrombosis of SMV
  - o Heparinize patients, rarely need surgery, only for resection of ischemic bowel

- What are characteristics of NOMI?
  - o Patients are generally critically ill, on multiple pressors and many times have cardiac failure
  - o Ischemia is in watershed areas (splenic flexure and upper rectum)
  - o Treatment is resuscitation and improvement of cardiac functions
  - o Only OR if need to resect ischemic bowel

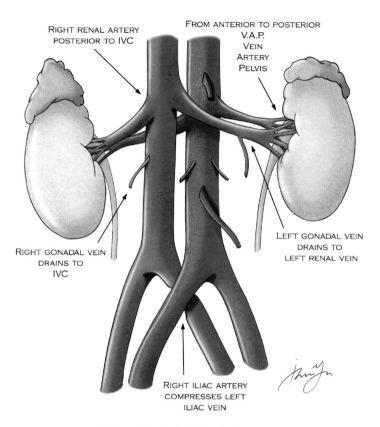

Figure 3. Abdominal Vascular Anatomy

Quick Hits

- What is most common site for a upper extremity embolus to lodge?

  o Brachial artery at bifurcation of radial and ulnar artery

- What is most common site for a lower extremity embolism to lodge

  o Common femoral artery at bifurcation of profunda and SFA

- In a patient with a ruptured AAA with hypotension that is getting a crash laparotomy. Where should you get proximal control?
  - Supraceliac aorta through the gastrohepatic ligament, underneath crus of diaphragm, press aorta against spine

- A patient that has a ruptured AAA that is being transferred to you, what do you tell the outside center to keep his BP at?
  - Permissive hypotension keep SBP 80-100

- MC organism in graft infections is?
  - Staph epidermidis (slow insidious bug)

- Treatment for popliteal entrapment syndrome?
  - Resect medial head of gastrocnemius

- What if a patient has refractory HTN and is found to have a beads on a string appearance in renal arteries or has same angiographic finding on internal carotids?
  - Fibromusclar dysplasia, most common in renal arteries and balloon angioplasty is treatment method of choice. Also seen in carotids

Aneurysms Continued...

- What is the most common splanchnic aneurysm and indications for operating on it?
  - Splenic artery
  - Operate on if >2 cm, or if pt is pregnant
  - Most can be coil embolized
  - If unstable perform splenectomy

- What is the clinical presentation of a ruptured splenic artery aneurysm?
  - "Double Rupture", due to containment by the lesser sac, and then free intraperitoneal rupture

- What size criteria should you treat hepatic and SMA aneurysms?

- o Treat when they reach 2 cm in size

- o Treat with resection and reconstruction

- What size criteria for treating iliac artery aneurysms?
  - o Commonly associated with abdominal aortic aneurysms

  - o 3.5 cm is size criteria for repair

  - o Generally repaired with endovascular stents

- What is the size criteria for treating femoral artery aneurysm, and what is most likely complication of femoral artery aneurysm?
  - o 2.5 historically but can be observed up to 3.5 cm

  - o Unlikely to rupture more likely to cause embolus or thrombosis

  - o Treat with resection and interposition

- Size criteria for treating popliteal artery aneurysms, what workup does patient need?
  - o 2 cm or if symptomatic (Embolic source or thrombosis)

  - o Pts need work up for AAA

- What are options for treating popliteal artery aneurysms
  - o Exclude and bypass or interposition with vein is the gold standard

  - o Endovascular stents are reasonable if patient is not a good candidate for open surgery

- Indications for operating on abdominal aortic aneurysms
  - o >5.5 cm in males or > 5 cm in females

  - o If growth > 1cm/year

  - o If symptomatic or infected (mycotic)

- When performing an open AAA repair when do you re-implant the IMA?
  - o If back pressure is poor or less than 40 mmHg

- If pulsatile back bleeding collateral flow is adequate, if minimal colon likely requires the additional flow from aorta

o If colon appears dusky or they had previous colonic surgery

- Disrupts collateral blood flow such as Arc of Riolan or Marginal Artery of Drummond

> Recognizing and managing complications is the most important aspect for ABSITE and oral boards.

- What vein is at risk for injury in an open AAA when clamping aorta proximally?
  o A retro-aortic left renal vein can be injured and cause significant bleeding
  o Important to evaluate for this on preoperative imaging

- Patient develops painless abdominal distention after starting a diet following an open AAA repair. Fluid is seen and tapped and noted to be milky, what is this condition called and how do you treat?
  o Chylous Ascites
  o Low fat, high protein diet with medium-chain fatty acid supplementation

- A patient after an open AAA repair develops abdominal pain and bloody diarrhea. What are you concerned for and what is algorithm to treat this condition?
  o Sigmoidoscopy to diagnose, along with starting IVF and IV abx
  o Many times can be managed nonoperatively, but if patients develop peritonitis, sepsis, or frankly necrotic colon seen on sigmoidoscopy they need an emergent colectomy with Hartman's pouch

- Which part of large intestine is spared from ischemia after AAA induced colonic ischemia
  o Middle and distal rectum as they have separate blood supply from sigmoid/upper rectum

- ○ Blood supply is from internal iliacs not IMA

- A pt is identified with a 4 cm abdominal aortic aneurysm how do you want to follow it
  - ○ Yearly duplex US if aneurysm is 4 cm or less
  - ○ If greater than 4 will need at least every 6 month duplex

- If you diagnose an infrarenal aortic graft infection, what is treatment of choice?
  - ○ -Axillary to bi-femoral bypass with aortic graft excision

- When you perform an aorto-bifemoral bypass how do you decide between end to end aortic anastomosis vs end to side anastomosis?
  - ○ Need to ensure flow into at least 1 internal iliac for pelvic perfusion
  - ○ If external iliacs are patent can perform end-end as patient will have internal iliac perfusion from retrograde flow
  - ○ If external iliacs are not patent can perform end-side anastomosis which will allow antegrade flow into internal iliacs assuming common iliacs are patent

- What anatomic criteria are needed to perform an EVAR?
  - ○ Neck diameter less than 32 mm
  - ○ A neck angle less than 60 degrees
  - ○ A neck length of at least 10 mm
  - ○ Iliac diameters of at least 7 mm
  - ○ Lack of thrombus or calcification in infrarenal neck

- What are the types of endoleaks and treatment options for each
  - ○ Type 1 (a proximal, b for distal)
    - Means the endograft isn't sealed at proximal or distal end point
    - These must be fixed, as risk of rupture
    - Generally place a cuff to seal more proximally or distally

- o Type II
    - Lumbars or IMA continue to fill aneurysm sac
    - Only need to be fixed if aneurysm sac continues to grow
    - Coil embolization of lumbars feeding sac is best treatment option
- o Type III
    - Components of the endograft are not sealed
    - Must be fixed, as aneurysm sac will be pressurized
    - Reinforce with cuff across previous interlap between components
- o Type IV
    - Porosity of graft, or a tear in the graft
    - May need to reline the graft with new endograft

Peripheral Vascular Disease

- How do you calculate an ABI?
    - o Take which ever pedal pressure is the highest (DP or PT) and divide that by the highest brachial pulse (right or left arm)

- How to interpret an ABI?
    - o .9 → 1.4 is normal

        .5 → .89 may have claudication

        <0.5 = May have rest pain

        <0.3 = Tissue loss

- What if patient has non compressible vessels, can you rely on ABIs?
    - o No small vessel calcification will lead to falsely elevated ABIs
    - o Toes pressures should be obtained, as these vessels are generally free from calcification

- A patient presents with claudication, how do you treat them?
  - Smoking cessation, exercise, statin therapy

- What indications would you intervene on a patient with claudication
  - Lifestyle limiting claudication that failed improvement with medical management
  - Tissue loss
  - Rest pain

 High yield! Do not offer operation for claudication, unless failed medical management and severe lifestyle impairment

- What options are there for imaging blood vessels
  - CTA is good for proximal vessels to level of knee if kidney function ok
  - If not angiography can use less contrast and visualize tibial vessels better
  - Also can do C02 angiography if very poor renal function
  - MRA is also an option

- What are essentials of operative planning in vascular surgery?
  - Inflow, outflow and vascular conduit (if bypass)

- What are principles of deciding between treating a lesion endovascular vs open
  - In general, endovascular interventions are best suited for lesions that are short and not heavily calcified.
  - Long occlusions that are densely calcified with good inflow, outflow and conduit are likely better treated with open bypass vs endarterectomy.
  - The common femoral artery is rarely treated with an endovascular approach because it is a mobile area that is prone to kinking and also because of the relative ease of an open approach.

- A patient presents with buttock claudication, impotence, and absence of femoral pulses, what is this syndrome called and where would you expect the lesions to be?
  - Leriche Syndrome
  - Aorto-iliac symptoms
  - Patient likely needs an aorto-bifemoral bypass

- If a patient presents with a large acute embolus that lodges at the aortic bifurcation, how does this differ in regards to treatment options compared to Leriche Syndrome?
  - Embolic disease can be treated with bilateral transfemoral retrograde embolectomy
  - Leriche syndrome is an atherosclerotic disease process for which a bypass would be indicated

- A pt presents with thigh claudication, where would you expect the lesion to be?
  - Iliac lesion

- A pt presents with calf claudication, where would you expect this lesion to be?
  - SFA

- Know basic anatomy of angiogram
  - You will have your anterior tibial artery branching first and going through intermuscular septum, you will then have tibial peroneal trunk, with peroneal coursing posterior to fibula, and posterior tibial doing just that, traveling behind the tibia

- What are the four compartments of the lower leg? And what do they contain
  - Anterior and lateral released with lateral fasciotomy incision
    - Anterior contains anterior tibial artery
    - Lateral compartment contains superficial peroneal nerve
  - Superficial and deep posterior
    - Superficial contains the gastrocnemius and sural nerve
    - Deep contains the tibial nerve, posterior tibial artery, and peroneal artery

- o What vessels does diabetes damage?

  - • Tibial vessels and small vessels of the feet

- In a patient with a diabetic foot wound, what imaging modality is the most sensitive for osteomyelitis?

  o MRI

- How to manage a diabetic foot ulcer with osteomyelitis in underlying bone?
  o Debride to healthy bone and then prolonged antibiotics 4-6 weeks.

- In any patient with a foot wound it is important to make sure adequate perfusion, how is this done
  o Start with non invasive flow studies (NIFs) and ABIs

  o If these show flow that is impaired the patient needs an angiogram that can be both diagnostic and therapeutic

Venous Disease

- How do operatively approach the left common iliac vein
  o By dividing the overlying right iliac artery, if the vein needs to be accessed and repaired

- What veins can be ligated in trauma
  o Can ligate any vein distal to renal veins

  o The closer to the renal veins the more morbidity, but if it is for exsanguinating hemorrhage it can be considered

  o If major vein ligation consider prophylactic fasciotomy

- Can you divide either renal vein?
  o You can divide the left renal vein if it is proximal to gonadal vein and gonadal vein is intact to allow retrograde drainage

DVT Management

- A pt has a swollen blue leg up to the buttocks, with motor and sensation intact, what are you worried about and what is the treatment?
  - Ileofemoral DVT causing phlegmasia cerulea dolens
  - Catheter directed thrombolysis is the treatment

- What is the most common location of DVTs? Which leg has a higher rate?
  - Ileofemoral DVTs are most common
  - Left leg is 2x more common than right

- Where should an IVC filter be placed in relation to the renal veins
  - Distal (caudad) to the renal veins

- How to long anticoagulate after a DVT
  - Provoked DVT = 3 months of therapy
  - Active Cancer = Continue therapy until no longer have cancer/cured
  - Hypercoaguable disorder = lifelong therapy

Quick Hits

- How to access SMA in trauma?
  - Exposure to SMA is by lifting of transverse colon and mobilizing ligament of treitz

- How to expose supraceliac aorta in trauma?
  - Enter lesser sac through gastrohepatic ligament, can divide posterior crus of diaphragm

- What is the biggest risk factor for ischemic colitis in a patient with a ruptured aneurysm?
  - Preoperative hypotension

- Old lady with headaches, and temporal blindness and fatigue, what is it and how do you treat?

- ○ Temporal arteritis
- ○ Diagnose with a temporal biopsy
- ○ Treat with corticosteroids

- What vessels are effected in Buerger's disease?
  - ○ Small to medium sized vessels

- Mycotic aneurysms what is the most common organism?
  - ○ Staphylococcus (not salmonella)

12 BREAST

High Yield Anatomy

- What are the surgical boundaries of the axillary lymph nodes?
  - o Level I – Lateral to pec minor
  - o Level II – Posterior to pec minor
  - o Level III – Medial to pec minor

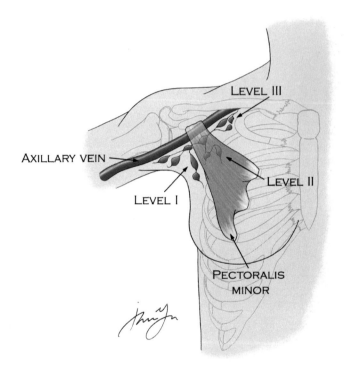

Figure 1. Surgical Levels of The Axillary Lymph Nodes

- Name the nerve that can be injured during an axillary dissection based on the clinical sequela
  - o Results in winged scapula:
    - Long thoracic innervating the serratus anterior
  - o Results in weakness in pullups and arm adduction:
    - Thoracodorsal nerve innervating the latissimus dorsi

- This nerve results in sensory deficits to the medial arm:
  - Intercostobrachial
- What nerve innervates both pec major and pec minor:
  - Medial pectoral nerve
  - Lateral pectoral nerve only innervates pec major

Lateral pectoral nerve only innervates pec major

- What is the blood supply to the breast?
  - Internal thoracic (aka mammary)
  - Intercostals
  - Lateral thoracic
  - Thoracoacromial arteries
- What is Batson's plexus?
  - Valveless venous plexus that allows direct hematogenous spread to the spine

Benign Breast Disease

- Breast Pain
  - Common, self-limited in most cases
  - Most frequent during the late luteal phase of the menstrual cycle
  - Treatment
    - Reassurance
    - For severe pain, the following have been studied with variable results:
      - danazol, bromocriptine, tamoxifen, primrose oil, vitamin E
- What is Mondor's disease and what is the treatment?
  - Superficial thrombophlebitis of the lateral thoracic vein or a tributary

- MC secondary to recent surgery, trauma, or other inflammatory process
- Rarely associated with carcinoma
  - o Presentation: tender, palpable subcutaneous cord
  - o Treatment: NSAIDs

- Fibrocystic disease
  - o Most common in perimenopausal women
  - o Symptoms: breast pain, nipple discharge, lumps that vary throughout menstrual cycle
  - o Treatment:
    - Simple cysts → observe
    - Symptomatic → aspirate
      - If aspirate is bloody or recurrent → cytology
      - Bloody aspirate → surgical excision
      - Unresolved after aspiration → surgical excision
      - Recurrence → surgical excision
  - o Is there a risk of cancer?
    - If cytology demonstrates atypical ductal or lobular hyperplasia

- Fibroadenoma and Phyllodes tumors
  - o Presentation: dominant mass
  - o Dx:
    - Imaging
      - If <35 yo → ultrasound (density of breast tissue)
      - If >35 yo → mammography
    - If findings are consistent with a benign fibroadenoma AND no risk factors → bi-annual ultrasound
    - If any uncertainty → core needle biopsy (CNB)
    - What if the mass continues to enlarge?
      - Need excisional biopsy
  - o Fibroadenoma variants

- Giant fibroadenoma
  - >6 cm, can be difficult to distinguish from phyllodes tumor
- Complex fibroadenoma = risk for developing carcinoma
  - Fibroadenoma with sclerosing adenosis, papillary apocrine hyperplasia, cysts, or epithelial calcifications
- Tubular adenoma = benign
  - Variant of peri canalicular fibroadenoma with adenosis-like epithelial proliferation
- o Phyllodes tumor
  - Subclassifications: benign, borderline, malignant
  - 10% become malignant (greater potential if >5 mitoses per high power field)
- o Rare hematogenous metastasis (does not go to nodes, so no sentinel lymph node biopsy (SLN) or Axillary dissection)
  - Treatment: Wide local excision (1 cm margins)
    - Do you need to perform SLN or axillary dissection?
      - o No. Hematogenous metastasis (rare)
- Nipple discharge
  - o What is the MC cause of bloody nipple discharge?
    - Intraductal papilloma (not premalignant)
  - o What findings are more concerning for malignancy?
    - Bloody, spontaneous, persistent, unilateral
    - <40 yo → 3% associated with cancer
    - >60 yo → 32% associated with malignancy
  - o Diagnosis:
    - Ductal fluid cytology, contrast ductogram, ductoscopy – minimally helpful
    - Best diagnostic test = Duct excision
  - o Treatment: subareolar resection of involved duct and papilloma

- Duct Ectasia
  - Dilation of the subareolar duct in peri- and post- menopausal women
  - Symptoms: cheesy, viscous nipple discharge
  - Treatment:
    - Asymptomatic → observe
    - Symptomatic → duct excision

- Breast Infections
  - What are the most common bacteria to cause both breast abscesses and mastitis?
    - Staphylococcus aureus
  - 2 groups:
    - Lactational - Most likely from blockage of the lactiferous ducts
      - If no abscess → antibiotics alone, continue breastfeeding
      - If abscess → aspiration and antibiotics, continue breastfeeding
        - I&D if does not resolve promptly
          - AE = concern for development of milk fistula
    - Nonlactational – Periductal infections associated with smoking and ductal ectasia
      - Tx: antibiotics, I&D if abscess present
  - Patient presents with recurrent, unresolving mastitis. What else do you need to do?
    - Biopsy of the skin to rule out inflammatory breast cancer

- Sclerosing Adenosis
  - Presentation: microcalcifications
  - Diagnosis: core needle biopsy
  - Treatment: if no atypia and concordant with imaging → observe

o Not a precursor to cancer

- Radial Scar
  - o Alternate names: sclerosing papillary proliferations, benign sclerosing ductal proliferation
  - o Diagnosis: mammogram – appears similar to small, invasive cancer
  - o Treatment: excisional biopsy
    - Associated with a small increased risk of cancer and the difference between invasive breast carcinoma may be difficult to determine on core biopsy alone

High Risk Breast Lesions

- Atypical lobular hyperplasia (ALH)
  - o Less well developed but morphologically similar to LCIS
  - o Not pre-malignant, but marker of increased risk
    - 8-12-fold greater lifetime risk, or ~1% per year
  - o Diagnosis: CNB
  - o Treatment: excisional biopsy
    - Why excise if not pre-malignant?
      - Discordant finding as these lesions are often incidental to the radiographic abnormality that prompted the biopsy

- Atypical ductal hyperplasia (ADH)
  - o Associated with a 4-5-fold increased risk of invasive cancer
  - o Diagnosis: CNB
  - o Treatment: Excisional biopsy
    - 9-30% incidence of DCIS on excisional biopsy
    - 3% chance of invasive ductal carcinoma (IDC)

- Lobular carcinoma in situ (LCIS)
  - Multifocal and bilateral, genetic predisposition
  - 90% ER/PR+ and HER2-
  - What is the malignancy risk?
    - Marker for 40% risk of CA development in EITHER breast
  - What type of cancer do they develop?
    - Ductal carcinoma
  - Treatment:
    - Wire localized excision
    - What if there is a positive margin?
      - No re-excision, adjuvant hormonal therapy
  - Pleomorphic LCIS = variant that is treated like DCIS

 No re-excision needed for LCIS when margin comes back positive

- Ductal carcinoma in situ (DCIS)
  - Malignant cells of the ductal epithelium without invasion of the basement membrane (premalignant lesion)
  - What is the malignancy risk?
    - 50% in ipsilateral breast
    - 5% in contralateral breast
  - Presentation: majority are non-palpable
  - Diagnosis: Mammography, CNB
  - Treatment:
    - Breast conserving therapy (BCT) = lumpectomy (1 cm margins) with adjuvant radiation (XRT)
      - Post op whole breast XRT reduces risk of local recurrence by 50% but does not affect overall survival
    - Large, multiquadrant, or contraindication to BCT → simple mastectomy + SLN

- Up to 25% DCIS may show invasive component on final pathology, so SLN sampling required before removing all breast tissue
- Skin and nipple-sparing procedures with immediate reconstruction are options
- Adjuvant therapy
  - Premenopausal → tamoxifen
  - Postmenopausal → aromatase inhibitor (anastrazole)
- What is the most aggressive subtype of DCIS?
  - Comedo
    - Characterized by necrosis
    - Treatment: simple mastectomy + adjuvant hormone therapy

DCIS excision need 2mm margin

Breast Cancer

- Screening
  - When should you start screening mammography?
    - Low risk: Age 40 every 2-3 years → annually after age 50
    - High risk: 10 years before youngest age of diagnosis in first-degree relative
      - Hereditary disorders with increased risk: BRCA 1/2, Li-Fraumeni (p53), Cowden syndrome (PTEN), Peutz-Jeghers (STK11), CDH1
        - BRCA 1/2 mutations → 10-20-fold increased risk → 30-60% risk by age 60
        - Screening age 25 with annual mammogram AND MRI + pelvic exam and CA-125
  - Findings on mammography that are concerning for malignancy: irregular borders, spiculated, distortion of breast, or small/thin linear branching calcification
  - BIRADS classification

	Risk	Management
0	Incomplete	Further imaging
1	Negative	Routine follow-up
2	Benign	Routine follow-up
3	Probably Benign	6 month follow-up
4	Suspicious for Malignancy	Biopsy
5	Highly Suggestive of Malignancy	Biopsy
6	Biopsy-Confirmed Malignancy	Excision

- Gail Model
  - Prediction model that calculates a woman's risk of developing breast cancer within the next 5 years and within her lifetime.
  - Variables:
    - Age
    - Age at first period
    - Age at the time of the birth of a first child (or has not given birth)
    - Family history of breast cancer (mother, sister or daughter)
    - Number of past breast biopsies
    - Number of breast biopsies showing atypical hyperplasia
    - Race/ethnicity
  - <u>Underestimates</u> risk for patients with strong family history (BRCA), personal hx of DCIS, LCIS, or invasive CA

- Invasive breast cancer
  - NCCN staging pearls

T1	0-2 cm	N1	1-3 nodes
T2	2-5 cm	N2	4-9 nodes
T3	>5 cm	N3	$\geq$10 nodes or supra/ infraclavicular
T4	Chest wall or skin involvement		

Stage 1	Small tumor, no nodes (T1N0M0)	Surgery + Adjuvant chemoXRT if indicated
Stage 2	Larger tumor, minor nodal involvement (T3N0 or T2N1)	Surgery + Adjuvant chemoXRT if indicated
Stage 3a/3b	Local invasion or more nodes (T4N0 or T3N2)	Surgery first vs neoadjuvant therapy
Stage 3c	Clavicular nodes (Any T, N3, M0)	Neoadjuvant + surgery if responds
Stage 4	Distal mets	Definitive chemotherapy

- Categories of breast cancer
  - What is the most common type of breast cancer?
    - Ductal carcinoma
  - What type of breast cancer is less common and does not typically form calcifications?
    - Lobular
  - Which subtype has the worse prognosis?
    - Signet ring cells
  - Inflammatory breast cancer
    - What is the typical presentation?
      - Inflamed, angry breast that is erythematous and warm
      - Characterized by rapid diffuse involvement of entire breast with cutaneous erythema and peau d'orange changes in the breast skin
    - What is the hallmark biopsy result?
      - Dermal lymphatic invasion
    - Staging: T4d by definition = at least Stage IIIb
    - Treatment = Neoadjuvant chemotherapy → modified radical mastectomy → adjuvant chemoXRT
      - NO BCT

o What are you concerned about if a patient presents with eczematous changes with scaling and ulceration of the skin and nipple?

- Paget's disease
  - What are the hallmarks of this disease?
    o Cells with clear cytoplasm and enlarged nucleoli
    o Marker of underlying malignancy – DCIS or IDC (generally ER-/PR- and HER2+
  - Treatment = Mastectomy including nipple-areolar complex + SLN

o Breast CA in men

- <1% of breast CA, usually ductal
- Risk factors: family history, Klinefelter's, BRCA 2 (15% of breast CA in men)
- What is the procedure of choice for a male with breast cancer?
  - Modified radical mastectomy
- Usually poor prognosis due to late presentation (same prognosis as women at similar stages)

o Breast CA in pregnancy

- Treatment in 1st trimester = modified radical mastectomy
- Late 2nd and 3rd trimester = BCT is an option
  - SLN with modified isotope dosing, post-op chemotherapy, and post-delivery breast radiation

- Treatment Options
  o Breast conserving (BCT): lumpectomy + whole breast irradiation
    - "No ink on tumor" = negative lumpectomy margin
    - Contraindications
      - Absolute
        o Pregnant and would require radiation during pregnancy

- o Multi-centric disease
- o Positive pathologic margins after re-excision
- Relative – previous radiation, active connective tissue disease, tumors >5cm

 For lumpectomy only margin needed is no ink on tumor

- o Simple mastectomy
  - • BCT equivalent to simple mastectomy
- o Chemotherapy
  - • Who gets chemotherapy?
    - • For the ABSITE:
      - o Tumors >1cm
        - • Exception = hormone receptor positive, node negative tumors with favorable oncotype characteristics can receive postop hormonal therapy alone
      - o Positive nodes
      - o Triple negative tumors
  - • What is the most common chemotherapy regimen?
    - • TAC
      - o Taxane (Docetaxel) → AE = peripheral neuropathy
      - o Adriamycin (Doxorubicin) → AE = cardiomyopathy
      - o Cyclophosphamide → AE = Hemorrhagic cystitis
        - • Mesna reduces risk of hemorrhagic cystitis
  - • Who is a candidate for neoadjuvant chemotherapy?
    - • Locally advanced/inoperable tumors: inflammatory, N2/N3, T4
    - • If tumor is too large relative to rest of breast for BCT and patient desires BCT
- o Radiotherapy

- Whole breast irradiation decreases local recurrence and improves survival

  - After lumpectomy whole breast irradiation with boost to tumor bead is strongly recommended

- What are the indications for XRT after mastectomy?

  - Advanced nodal disease (>4 nodes), fixed nodes, internal mammary nodes

  - Skin/chest wall involvement

  - Positive margins

  - T3/T4 tumor, which is greater than 5cm

- Regional node irradiation

  - >4 positive lymph nodes → XRT to supraclavicular, infraclavicular, and axillary LN

  - Tumor central to inner area of breast → internal mammary node radiation

  - 1-3 positive LN → grey zone, depends on individual characteristics

- Radiation is given AFTER chemotherapy

- Radiation in older adults

  - NCCN guidelines allow for the use of lumpectomy with negative margins plus hormonal therapy WITHOUT radiation in women >70 with clinically negative nodes and ER+ T1 breast CA

o Endocrine therapy

  - For Estrogen/Progesterone receptor (ER/PR) positivity

  - Which has better prognosis receptor positive or receptor negative patients?

    - Receptor positive

    - More common in post-menopausal women

  - Which has the better prognosis, ER or PR+?

    - PR+

    - Both is even better!

- Treatment = 5 years of tamoxifen (pre-menopausal) or aromatase inhibitor (post-menopausal women)
  - HER2 targeted therapy
    - With HER2/neu receptor, is prognosis better or worse if positive?
      - Worse
    - Treatment = traztuzumab (Herceptin) for 1 year

- Axillary staging
  - What is the most prognostic factor in staging of breast cancer?
    - Nodal status
      - 0 positive nodes → 75% 5-year survival
      - 4-10 nodes → 40% 5-year survival
  - SLN indicated for all invasive tumors
    - ACOSOG Z0011 Trial = RCT comparing SLN to axillary dissection
      - Women > 18yo with T1/T2 tumors, <3 positive SLN, BCT + whole breast XRT
      - No difference in local recurrence, disease free survival, overall survival at median follow up of 6.3 years

> Z11 is critical especially for oral boards
> If T1-T2 with < 3 positive SLN
> AND patient is going to receive whole-breast radiation
> No benefit to axillary dissection

  - Axillary dissection recommended for:
    - Clinically positive nodes confirmed by FNA or CNB
    - Sentinel nodes not identified
    - What nodes do you take?
      - Level 1 and 2
    - What nodes do you take in an axillary dissection for melanoma?
      - Levels 1-3

Quick Hits

- Patient presents with a dominant breast mass. Next step?
  - IMAGING — Bilateral mammography and/or U/S

- Concerning lesion on mammography – core needle biopsy returns normal?
  - Excisional biopsy for discordant findings

- Most common sites for breast cancer metastases?
  - Bone, lung, brain, and liver
  - Isolated tumor cell deposits (<0.2mm) do NOT constitute metastatic disease

- Valveless venous system responsible for bony metastasis to spine?
  - Batson's plexus

- What is the cumulative risk of breast and ovarian CA with BRCA1 and BRCA2?
  - BRCA1 – 65% breast, 40% ovary
  - BRCA2 – 45% breast, 10% ovary

- Side effects of tamoxifen?
  - Thromboembolism
  - Increased risk of uterine CA

- Chronic lymphedema for 10 years following axillary dissection, now with dark purple lesion on upper arm?
  - Stewart-Treves Syndrome (lymphangiosarcoma)

- What is Poland's syndrome?
  - Hypoplasia of the chest wall, amastia, hypoplastic shoulder, no pectoralis muscle

- What are the nodes between the pectoralis major and minor called?
  - Rotter's nodes

13 HEMATOLOGY

- A patient with a platelet disorder will have what coagulation lab abnormality?
  - Increased bleeding time (PT and PTT not reliably affected)

- What is the most common congenital bleeding disorder? And what are the different types
  - Von Willebrand's Disease
    - Type I – Most common, reduced quantity of vWf, treat with desmopressin (for most patients) or cryoprecipitate
    - Type II – Dysfunctional vWF , treat with desmopressin or cryoprecipitate
    - Type III – Complete absence of vWF, desmopressin does not work, must use cryoprecipitate or Factor VIII replacement

- What bleeding disorders is cryoprecipitate helpful in?
  - Von Willebrand's, hypofibrinogenemia, hemophilia A

- What are the factors missing in Hemophilia A and Hemophilia B
  - Hemophilia A = Factor VIII, prolongation of PTT
    - Treat with factor VIII or cryo
  - Hemophilia B = Factor IX, prolongation of PTT
    - Treat with factor IX or FFP

- Coumadin = WEPT = Warfarin Extrinsic pathway PT

- PTT = intrinsic pathway

- A patient on coumadin undergoes surgery and following surgery platelets drop >50%, what tests to confirm the diagnosis? Treatment?
  - Concern for Heparin Induced Thrombocytopenia
  - Clinical suspicion with 4Ts score (thrombocytopenia, timing, thrombosis, and other possible causes)
  - ELISA testing anti-platelet-factor-4 for initial screening
  - Serotonin release assay for confirmation

- Stop heparin immediately with sufficient clinical suspicion
- Start safe anticoagulation (argatroban is classic; bivalirudin or fondaparinux also options)

- Patient presents with DVT and strong family history of DVT. What heritable blood clotting disorders would be on your differential?
  - Factor V Leiden
  - Prothrombin Gene Defect 20210
  - Protein C and S Deficiency
  - Antithrombin 3 Deficiency
  - Hyperhomocystenemia

- A patient is started on Coumadin and develops skin necrosis, what is the name of this phenomena and what is its pathophysiology?
  - Warfarin induced skin necrosis
  - Seen in patients with protein C and S deficiency
  - Short half-life of protein C and S (natural anticoagulants), leads to brief period of time where patient is hypercoagulable
  - Important to bridge with Lovenox when starting coumadin

- Patients with hyperhomocysteinemia, how to treat this?
  - Folic acid and B12

- How does antithrombin III deficiency present itself, and how do you treat it?
  - They do not respond to heparin
  - Treat with ATIII concentrate or FFP, prior to heparin admin
  - Then start on long-term anticoagulant

- Mechanism of action of heparin? And how to reverse?
  - Potentiates ATIII, makes it 1000x more potent
  - Protamine to reverse
    - Can cause hypotension and bradycardia

- What are characteristics of antiphospholipid syndrome, how do you diagnose and how do you treat it?
  - History – symptoms of Lupus, prior DVTs, or recurrent pregnancy losses
  - Will have prolonged PTT but are hypercoaguable
  - Caused by antibodies to cardiolipin and lupus anticoagulant
  - Treat with heparin bridge to coumadin

- What is mechanism of action of Warfarin?
  - Inhibits VKORC (a protein that reduces Vitamin K to activate it)
  - Inhibits creation of Factors X, IX, VII, II (1972) and protein and C and S
  - Contraindicated in pregnant patients

- Warfarin reversal agents and their times to onset
  - Administer Vit K (6 hours)
  - FFP (<1 hour)
  - Prothrombin Concentrate Complex (immediate)

- How do determine effectiveness of Lovenox
  - Check factor Xa levels
  - Unlike heparin, Lovenox is only weakly reversed by protamine

- Reversal agents for direct oral anticoagulants (DOACs)
  - Dabigatran (Pradaxa)
    - Can be reversed with dialysis
    - And idarucizumab (Praxbind; monoclonal Ab that inactivates it)
  - Apixaban (Eliquis) and rivaroxaban (Xarelto)
    - Can be reversed with andexanet alfa (Andexxa; decoy-receptor for factor Xa inhibitor molecules)

Anticoagulant	Half-life (hours)	Reversal
Coumadin/Warfarin	20 - 60	PCC (immediate) FFP (< 1 hr) Vitamin K (6 hrs)
Pradaxa/Dabigatran	12 - 17	Dialysis Praxbind (monoclonal ab)
Xarelto/Rivaroxaban	5 - 9	Andexxa (recombinant factor Xa)
Eliquis/Apixaban	12	Andexxa (recombinant factor Xa)
Unfractionated heparin (UFH)	1 - 1.5	Protamine sulfate
Lovenox/Enoxaparin	4.5 - 7	Protamine sulfate (less effective than with UFH)

- What is mechanism of action of tPA? How to reverse it?
  - Activates plasminogen, breaks down fibrinogen
  - Aminocaproic acid
- What are contraindications to using tPA?
  - Absolute
    - Active internal bleeding
    - Recent CVA or neurosurgery
    - Recent GI bleed, or intracranial pathology
  - Relative contraindications
    - Surgery past 10 days
    - Recent organ biopsies, recent delivery
    - Recent major trauma
    - Uncontrolled hypertension
- Which coagulation factors are not synthesized in the liver?
  - Factor VIII, and Desmopressin
- When to use FFP
  - FFP has all coagulation factors
  - Any coagulation disorder including Antithrombin III deficiency

- What factors are measured by PT/INR
  - Measures external pathway – factors II, VII, IX, X (1972)
  - Best test for liver synthetic function
  - Goal INR of 2-3 generally in anticoagulated patients
- What factors are measured by PTT
  - All except VII
  - Goal of 60-90 in anticoagulated patients

Quick Hits

- Thrombin (factor II) is key to coagulation
  - Fibrinogen to fibrin
  - Activates platelets
- Fibrin links platelets (GpIIb/IIIa molecules) to form a platelet plug
- Antithrombin III is key to anticoagulation
  - Binds and inhibits thrombin
  - Heparin activates AT-III
- What factors are made in liver?
  - All except VIII and vWF
- Factor with the shortest half-life
  - Factor VII
- What factors does warfarin block?
  - Vit K dependent factors: II, VII, IX, X, protein C and S
- What does cryo contain?
  - High concentrations of vWF, VIII, and fibrinogen
- What is in FFP
  - All clotting factors, some fibrinogen

14 TRAUMA

Initial Assessment

- Always start with ABCDE's (Primary Survey). A lot of trauma questions on the ABSITE just want you to be able to prioritize. Always address the airway first!!!
  - o Can't intubate, can't ventilate → Crichothyroidotomy (See Image)

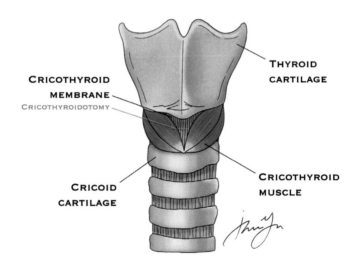

- Disability – Looking for signs of intracranial pressure, not meant to be a complete neurologic assessment. GCS and pupil exam are the most important factors.
  - o GCS – What component has the most prognostic ability?
    - Answer: Motor Score
  - o GCS < 8 → Intubate
  - o Pupillary Exam
    - Unilateral fixed dilated pupil → Ipsilateral space occupying lesion (blood) with compression of optic nerve
    - Bilateral pinpoint pupils → Pontine hemorrhage

Head Trauma

- Who needs an ICP Monitor?
  - GCS < 8 with abnormal head CT
  - 2 main types of ICP monitors: Ventriculostomy and "bolt"
    - Ventriculostomy – Drain placed in ventricle. Has the advantage of being able to drain CSF if needed to decrease ICP.
    - Bolt – Placed intraparenchymal.

- Golden Rule of Head Trauma = avoid hypotension and hypoxia to avoid secondary brain injury

- Cushing's Reflex – Bradycardia, Hypertension, Altered Respirations
  - Late finding, indicates impending herniation
  - Initial management – Elevate HOB, ventilate to pC02 35, Mannitol and/or Hypertonic Saline, Sedate and Paralyze

- Epidural Hematoma
  - Presentation: Hit in head, lucid interval followed by rapid GCS deterioration
  - Head CT shows lenticular lucency that is contained by suture lines

- Subdural Hematoma
  - Presentation: Older person on Coumadin with GLF
  - Crescent shaped lucency that crosses suture lines

- Intraparenchymal Hemorrhage (most common in trauma)
  - Common after blunt injury (e.g. MVC)

- Subarachnoid Hemorrhage
  - Worst headache of life, spontaneous

- Cerebral Perfusion Pressure (CPP) = MAP - ICP
  - CPP is surrogate for cerebral blood flow
  - Ideally keep CPP > 60 and ICP < 20

- o Main regulator of CPP?
  - PaCO2
- o In TBI, autoregulation is lost. Thus, CPP is exquisitely sensitive to changes in MAP.

- Interventions to reduce ICP
  - o Elevate head of bed
  - o Remove c-collar or anything around neck
  - o Hyperventilation (short term)
  - o Hypertonic Saline or Mannitol (Hypertonic saline preferred in trauma due to hypotension that can result from mannitol administration)
  - o Sedation/Paralysis

- Adjuncts in the treatment of head injury
  - o Seizure prophylaxis for trauma with intracranial bleed.
    - 1-week prophylaxis, prevents early seizures
  - o Early enteral feeding within 24-48hrs
  - o Correct coagulopathy
    - Reversal agents for coagulopathy
      - Coumadin -- PCC for rapid reversal. FFP is also okay. Add Vit K
      - Pradaxa (Dabigatran) – Dialysis or Praxbind (idarucizumab)
      - Apixaban/Rivaroxaban – PCC gives partial reversal
  - o What about Steroids?
    - No benefit and potential harm

Spine Trauma

- Who can be cleared clinically?
  - o No distracting injury
  - o GCS 15, non-intoxicated
  - o No midline tenderness, no neurologic deficits

- Radiographic clearance?
  - Generally, patients with a normal CT scan and no localizing symptoms can be cleared (somewhat controversial)
- Spinal cord injury syndromes
  - Central cord syndrome – Typically upper extremity weakness (cape and gloves
    - Generally elderly patient with spinal stenosis
  - Brown Sequard (hemi-section)
    - Ipsilateral motor deficit and contralateral pain/temperature deficit below level of injury
    - Generally, results from penetrating (stab) injury
  - Anterior cord syndrome
    - Motor deficit below level of injury
    - Results from vascular injury to anterior spinal artery
  - Spinal Cord Injury Without Radiographic Abnormality (SCIWORA)
    - Seen in pediatric population
- Neurogenic shock vs. Spinal Shock
  - Neurogenic shock
    - Affects hemodynamics. Hypotensive and Bradycardic.
  - Spinal Shock
    - Sensory/Motor affects. No effect on hemodynamics.
    - Absent bulbocavernosus and cremasteric reflex.
    - Some functions may return with spinal shock.
    - Intact reflexes indicate deficits are likely permanent.
- Management
  - No steroids for spinal injury
  - Stable vs unstable
    - `2 of 3 columns disrupted = unstable and requires operative fixation

Neck Trauma

- Zones of the neck
  - o Zone 1 – clavicles to cricoid cartilage
  - o Zone 2 – cricoid cartilage to the angle of the mandible
  - o Zone 3 – Angle of mandible to skull base

- Penetrating neck injury and patient hypotensive → OR

- Penetrating neck injury with hard sign of vascular injury → OR

- Penetrating neck injury and patient stable without hard sign of vascular injury → CT neck including CT angiogram
  - o If concerned for esophageal injury → add esophagram or EGD

- Esophageal injury
  - o Extend myotomy to see mucosal injury extent, repair in 2 layers, buttress, drain
  - o Can't locate injury during neck exploration → widely drain

- Blunt cerebrovascular injury (BCVI)
  - o Consider screening imaging (CTA) for:
    - Severe cervical hyperextension/rotation or hyperflexion mechanism
    - Hanging mechanism
    - Neurological examination not explained by brain imaging
    - Diffuse axonal injury
    - Skull base fractures involving the foramen lacerum
    - Horner's syndrome
    - LeFort II or III facial fractures
    - Cervical spine fracture, particularly C1-C3
    - Epistaxis from a suspected arterial source after trauma
    - Blunt head trauma with GCS < 8
    - Cervical bruit, hematoma
    - An isolated cervical seat belt sign without other risk factors

and normal physical examination has failed to be identified as an independent risk factor in two retrospective studies and should not be used as the sole criteria to stratify patients for screening.

o Distal internal carotid is most common site for BCVI

o Antiplatelet therapy is generally treatment for most BCVI

o Endovascular intervention for pseudoaneurysm of AV fistula

Thoracic Trauma

• Indications for OR following thoracic trauma based on chest tube output
    o Controversial and data limited
    o In general, for boards to OR if:
        • >1500ml output after initial placement
        • 200ml/hr output over 4 hours

• Flail Chest – 3 consecutive rib fractures in 2 locations
    o Cause of hypoxia with flail chest → underlying pulmonary contusion
    o Management:
        • Pain control (epidural)
        • Consider PPV, rib plating

• Sternal fracture
    o Be concerned about blunt cardiac injury
    o EKG is required for all suspected blunt cardiac injuries → Sinus tach and PVCs are the most common abnormalities
    o Utility of Troponin as screening tool for BCVI is controversial -- However, a normal ECG and normal Troponin essentially rule out blunt cardiac injury
    o If patient demonstrated hemodynamic instability or persistent new arrhythmia → Echocardiogram

• Blunt Aortic injury (BAI)
    o The proximal descending aorta, where the relatively mobile

aortic arch can move against the fixed descending aorta (ligamentum arteriosum), is at greatest risk from the shearing forces of sudden deceleration, although other segments or vessels can be affected.

o Physical exam – Hypotension, upper extremity hypertension, unequal blood pressures, external evidence of major chest trauma, thoracic outlet hematoma, fractured sternum, fractured thoracic spine, left flail chest

o Must maintain a high index of suspicion based on mechanism of injury or initial imaging

o CXR has low sensitivity – However, findings concerning for BAI include 1) widened mediastinum (8cm), 2) Depression of mainstem bronchus, 3) deviation of NG tube to the right, 4) Apical Cap, Disruption of calcium ring (broken halo)

- In short –Any clinical suspicion based on mechanism or a "funny looking" mediastinum on CXR needs further imaging

- CT angiography of the chest is comparable with aortography and is the diagnostic study of choice

o Classification scheme for grading the severity of aortic injury

- Type I (intimal tear)

- Type II (intramural hematoma)

- Type III (pseudoaneurysm)

- Type IV (rupture)

o Management

- Patients should be immediately started on anti-hypertensive regimens to maintain systolic blood pressure within a "normal" range, generally less that 120mm Hg (B-Blocker, typically esmolol, with or without nitroprusside)

- Most blunt aortic injuries surviving to hospital are partial-transections, and should be managed with blood pressure control until the definitive repair.

  - Thus, the priority in the management of hemodynamically unstable patients with potential aortic injury is to rapidly identify and control on-going hemorrhage from other sites, and to avoid over-resuscitation.

- In patients diagnosed with BAI, it is strongly recommended to use of endovascular repair over open repair

o Post endovascular repair of BAI develops left hand ischemia?

- Patient needs Carotid to subclavian bypass (subclavian is covered routinely during endovascular repair of BAI)

Abdominal Trauma

- Blunt Abdominal Trauma

o Focused Abdominal Sonography for Trauma (FAST) exam -- Only looking for free fluid in abdomen or pericardium

- Fluid = blood, succus, or urine

- CT scan is more sensitive/specific than FAST

- FAST can have false negative – should be repeated in unstable patients

o Most common injuries following blunt abdominal trauma -- Solid organ injury

- Hollow viscus or pancreas are the most commonly missed injury

o Abdominal seat belt sign – Should be concerned for bowel injury or pancreatic injury

o Solid organ injury and hemodynamically unstable → OR

o Solid organ injury and hemodynamically stable → Generally non-operative management – ICU monitoring, trend labs, supportive care

- Take to OR for ongoing transfusion requirement or if patient becomes unstable

o CT scan with free fluid and no solid organ injury → Hollow viscus injury until proven otherwise

o Hemodynamically stable with blush on CT (Spleen, liver, kidney) → Angioembolization

- Abdominal stab wounds
  - o Work-up and Management
    - Hemodynamically unstable, evisceration, peritoneal signs → OR
    - Anterior stab wounds
      - Local wound exploration
        - o Look for violation of **anterior rectus sheath**.
          - If truly negative and no other injuries – Can discharge patient
          - If violation of anterior sheath:
          - Can observe with serial exams if hemodynamically stable and examinable +/- CT
          - If hemodynamically stable and unexaminable → CT vs laparoscopic exploration looking for violation of posterior fascia/peritoneum (controversial)
    - Flank stab wounds
      - Concerned about retroperitoneal structures
      - Triple contrast CT scan – Oral, Rectal, and IV
    - Thoracoabdominal Stab wound
      - Be concerned for diaphragm injury, even if completely stable and negative imaging
        - o Frequently missed on CT -- Best evaluated with laparoscopy
- Bowel injury
  - o Destructive = >50% circumference bowel wall involvement or devascularized
    - Treatment: Resection and anastomosis
  - o Non-Destructive = <50% and no vascular compromise
    - Treatment: Primary Repair
  - o Damage control setting with destructive bowel injury
    - Staple off bowel, leave in discontinuity (No anastomosis),

temporary abdominal closure, and take to ICU for resuscitation

- o Penetrating Colon Injury

  - • Treatment: Primary repair for non-destructive injury; Resection and anastomosis for destructive injury

  - • Old teaching was a diversion for left-sided injury. Decision to divert is now based more on patients' physiologic status. Left-sided injury no longer mandates diversion.

- o Bucket Handle Injury

  - • Typically from blunt injury

  - • Mesentery of bowel in torn from bowel but bowel intact

  - • Treatment: Resection

- • Pancreatic Injury

  - o Key factors for management: Involvement of pancreatic duct, Location (Head, Body, or Tail), associated duodenal injury

  - o Distal injury with no ductal injury → Leave drains

  - o Distal injury with duct injury → Distal pancreatectomy with splenectomy

    - • Can consider spleen sparing in hemodynamically stable children

  - o Laceration to head of pancreas with or without ductal injury → Drainage only

- • Retroperitoneal Hematoma

  - o Zone 1 – Central (aorta, vena cava)

  - o Zone 2 – Lateral (renal)

  - o Zone 3 – Pelvis (Iliac)

  - o Penetrating injury – explore all 3

  - o Blunt Injury

    - • Zone 1 – explore

    - • Zone 2 – explore only expanding/pulsatile hematoma

    - • Zone 3 – Generally don't explore (pack and angiography)

- Pelvic Fracture
  - o Be concerned about injury to adjacent structures (rectum, bladder, vagina, urethra)
  - o Open book pelvic fracture with hypotension → Pelvic binder 1st step
    - Angiography in stable patient
    - OR for Preperitoneal packing in unstable patient

Shock

- Shock is defined as "end organ hypoperfusion"
- Classes of Hemorrhage
  - o Class I = 0-15% blood loss
    - Generally, no physiologic signs
  - o Class II = 15-30% blood loss
    - Tachycardia, Narrowed pulse pressure
  - o Class III = 30-40% blood loss
    - Hypotension
  - o Class IV = >40% blood loss
- Earliest sign of shock: Tachycardia and narrowed pulse pressure (Class II)
- Triad of death: Hypothermia, Coagulopathy, Acidosis
- Damage control principles: Control sepsis/spillage and hemorrhage, temporary closure, and resuscitate
  - o Return to OR when physiologically corrected
- Abdominal Compartment Syndrome
  - o 1st signs: Increased peak pressures on vent, decreased Up
  - o Confirm with bladder pressure
    - Absolute pressure >20 is concerning for ACS
  - o Treatment is decompressive laparotomy
    - Be cautious about decompressive laparotomy in burn patients following massive resuscitation as it is associated

with high mortality. In burn patients, drain placement to drain ascites for ACS is preferred.

- Damage Control Resuscitation
  - Avoid crystalloid if at all possible. Key is permissive hypotension.
  - Balanced blood product resuscitation of platelets, PRBC, and FFP in a 1:1:1 ratio
  - Bleeding trauma patient requiring massive blood product resuscitation
    - Give TXA – 1g within 3 hours of injury with subsequent 1g given over 8 hours
      - Decreases fibrinolysis
    - Answer is NEVER Factor VII – No longer given in trauma
    - TEG/ROTEM can guide resuscitation if available. Used more and more and may start showing up on ABSITE/ Boards (See Image).
      - Time – How long it takes to start clot
        - If prolonged → Give FFP
      - Angle – How fast they are forming a strong clot
        - If low → Give Cryoprecipitate
      - Amplitude – Size of clot
        - If low → Platelets
      - LY30 – Measure Lysis
        - If high → Give TXA

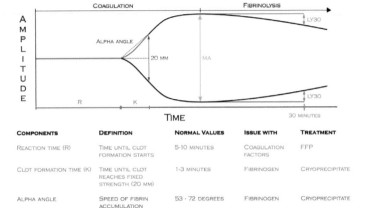

COMPONENTS	DEFINITION	NORMAL VALUES	ISSUE WITH	TREATMENT
REACTION TIME (R)	TIME UNTIL CLOT FORMATION STARTS	5-10 MINUTES	COAGULATION FACTORS	FFP
CLOT FORMATION TIME (K)	TIME UNTIL CLOT REACHES FIXED STRENGTH (20 MM)	1-3 MINUTES	FIBRINOGEN	CRYOPRECIPITATE
ALPHA ANGLE	SPEED OF FIBRIN ACCUMULATION	53 - 72 DEGREES	FIBRINOGEN	CRYOPRECIPITATE
MAXIMUM AMPLITUDE (MA)	HIGHEST AMPLITUDE	50 - 70 MM	PLATELETS	PLATELETS/DDAVP
LYSIS AT 30 MINUTES (LY30)	PERCENTAGE OF AMPLITUTDE LOSS 30 MINUTES AFTER MA	0 - 8%	EXCESS FIBRINOLYSIS	TRANEXEMIC ACID/ AMINOCAPROIC ACID

Urologic Trauma

- Bladder Injury
  - Frequently associated with pelvic fractures
  - Will always have hematuria (Renal injury may not have hematuria)
  - Management:
    - Intraperitoneal injury → Operative repair
    - Extraperitoneal injury → Foley drainage

- Ureteral Injury
  - Management
    - Mid Ureteral Injury – spatulate ends, primary anastomosis over double J stent with fine absorbable suture
    - Distal Ureteral Injury– Re-implant into bladder.
      - If it doesn't reach?
        - Psoas Hitch

- Urethra Injury
  - Physical Exam – Blood at meatus, scrotal/perineal hematoma, high riding prostate
  - Diagnosis – Retrograde Urethrogram.

Extremity Trauma

- Hard signs of vascular injury
  - Pulsatile bleeding, expanding hematoma, absent pulses, bruit/thrill
- Soft signs
  - Non-expanding hematoma, decreased pulses (ABI <0.9), proximity to neurovascular structures
- Soft signs of injury → CT angiogram
- Extremity arterial trauma – Generally answer is repair with reversed saphenous
- Extremity venous injury – Generally primary repair if possible or simply ligate
- Popliteal artery and vein → Don't forget to add fasciotomy after repair

Special Populations Pearls

- Pediatric Trauma Patients
  - Airway
    - Airway is narrow, short, and more anterior than in adults
    - Intubate with cuffed tubed (recently changed dogma)
      - uncuffed tube in infants only
    - ET tube size
      - Size of patient's pinky nail bed width
      - Age/4 + 4 = ET tube size
    - Bradycardia is common with direct laryngoscopy → Have atropine ready
  - 20cc/kg bolus for crystalloid; 10cc/kg bolus for blood

products

- Pregnant Trauma Patients
  - o Physiologic changes in pregnancy
    - Increase in circulating blood volume with physiological dilution/anemia
    - Increased respirations, decreased tidal volume results in respiratory alkalosis
  - o Place patient left side down to take pressure off IVC
  - o Abdominal trauma in pregnant patient
    - Be concern for placental abruption and maternal-fetal hemorrhage
      - Give RhoGAM if mother Rh- if concern for maternal-fetal hemorrhage
        - o Kleihauer Betke Test can be used – looks for fetal blood cells in maternal circulation
  - o Who needs fetal monitoring?
    - For viable pregnancies → Generally 24weeks gestation or greater

Quick Hits

- Bubbles seen in Coronary vessels during resuscitative thoracotomy?
  - o Air embolism, typically from pulmonary injury

- MVC with lumbar chance fracture and seat belt sign?
  - o Hollow viscus injury, maybe pancreatic injury

- Kid with handle bar blow to abdomen?
  - o Duodenal hematoma

- Left thoracoabdominal stab injury with negative imaging and normal exam?
  - o Laparoscopy looking for diaphragm injury

- Posterior knee dislocation?

- o Popliteal artery injury

- Patient found down, oliguric, Cr 3.5?
  - o Rhabdomyolysis

- Tracheostomy patient and nurse reports 10cc of bright red blood from tracheostomy site
  - o Tracheoinnominate fistula with sentinel bleed

- Severe TBI patient with Na 155 and 5L Up?
  - o Diabetes insipidus
  - o Treatment? → DDAVP

- Trauma patient paralyzed from head down with no cremasteric reflex?
  - o Spinal shock

- Stab wound to abdomen, benign exam, eviscerated omentum?
  - o Laparotomy

- Liver bleeding unchanged after Pringle maneuver?
  - o Hepatic Vein or retrohepatic vena cava injury

- Chest x-ray with apical cap?
  - o Blunt thoracic aortic injury

- Major arterial bleeding posterior in neck exploration?
  - o Vertebral artery injury

- Stab wound to flank?
  - o Kidney or colon injury, hence need for triple contrast CT

- Trauma patient with elevated LY30 on TEG?
  - o Give TXA

- Gateway structure to carotid bifurcation?
  - o Common facial vein

- Gateway structure for great vessels during median sternotomy?
  - o Innominate Vein

- Hematemesis 2 weeks after MVC with Grade IV liver laceration.
  - Haemobilia
  - Treatment? → angioembolization

- Open pelvic fracture with complex perineal wound?
  - Diverting colostomy

- GSW to pelvis with rectal wall hematoma seen on rigid proctoscopy?
  - Diverting colostomy

15 CRITICAL CARE

Ventilator Settings and Management

- Most physiologic ventilator mode?
  - o Iron lung (Negative Pressure Ventilation)

- Ventilator induced lung injury
  - o Volume
  - o Pressure (Barotrauma)
  - o Oxygen Toxicity

- Oxygenation vs Ventilation
  - o Oxygenation affected by:
  - o Fi02, PEEP, Mean Airway Pressure
  - o Ventilation affected by:
  - o RR, Tidal Volume
  - o RR x TV = Minute Ventilation

- Peak pressure – reflects pressure in large airways

- Plateau pressure – must do inspiratory pause. This allows pressures to equilibrate and better reflects alveolar pressure

- What if there is large differential between peak and plateau pressure (e.g. Peak 50, Plateau 30)?
  - o Large airway obstruction
  - o Bronchospasm

- What if peak and plateau are both high?
  - o Alveolar lung disease (e.g. ARDS)

- Negative inspiratory Force (NIF) – Must do expiratory pause to check this.

- Vent Modes
  - o Continuous mandatory ventilation (CMV)/Assist Control (AC)
    - Respiratory Rate (RR) and Volume are set
    - Every breath is fully supported
    - Problems: Volume is set regardless of pressure and can result in barotrauma; hyperventilation if patient RR is high.

- o Pressure Support (PS)
  - Pressure is set
  - Advantages: Limits barotrauma
  - Disadvantages: Hypoventilation
- o Synchronized Intermittent Mandatory Ventilations (SIMV)
  - RR and Volume set
  - Spontaneous breaths above set rate are not fully supported
  - Delivered breaths are synchronized – typically a more comfortable mode of breathing
  - Problems: Patients can tire out
- o Extubation criteria
- o Spontaneous Breathing Trial (SBT) should be done every day
- o Follows commands (i.e. neurologically able to protect airway)
- o Minimal Vent Settings for extubation (in general):
  - Fi02 50% or less
  - PEEP <10
  - Rapid shallow RR/TV < 100 (Best Predictor)
  - NIF > 20 (Good predictor of who will fail if <20; However >20 is poorly predictive of who will do well)

Acute Respiratory Distress Syndrome (ARDS)

- Definition: Within 1 week of insult, characteristic radiographic finding, not cardiogenic
  - o Mild: P:F ratio = 200-300
  - o Moderate: P:F ratio = 100-200
  - o Severe: P:F ratio = <100
- Ventilator strategies for ARDS
  - o Lung protection ARDSNET protocol – Low tidal volume (4-6cc/kg)

o Permissive hypercapnia

- Generally, as long as pH above 7.20 it is recommended to allow hypercapnia as long as the patient is oxygenating. This avoids further lung injury.

o Strategies for ARDS patients that are failing

- Airway Pressure Release Ventilation (APRV)

  - Long inhalation period with short extubation

  - Set P-high (Pressure High) and P-Low (Pressure Low) as well as T-high (Time High) and T-Low (Time Low)

    o Want long T-high and short T-low

  - Patient can breathe spontaneously throughout

  - Proning

  - Nitrous Oxide, NM blockade

  - Proning and neuromuscular blockade have proven benefits for ARDS in prospective RCTs

Sepsis

- Old definition – Focused on inflammation (SIRS Criteria)
  o Sepsis = SIRS + infection source

  o Severe Sepsis = SIRS + source + end organ dysfunction

  o Septic Shock = SIRS + end organ dysfunction + hypotension/pressor requirement

  o New Definition – Focuses more on organ dysfunction with infection (SOFA Score)

  o SOFA = Sequential Organ Function Assessment

  o Sepsis = If SOFA score increases by 2 or more points, or a score of 2 or more on a patient initial presentation

  o Septic Shock = Pressor requirement AND lactate of 2 or more despite resuscitation

- Diagnostic adjuncts
  o Procalcitonin – when normalizes can be a guide to stop antibiotics

- Better at ruling out sepsis if negative; More sensitive than specific
  - o 1,3 beta-d-glucan assay for fungal infections
  - o Mannan antigen and anti-mannan antibody for invasive candidiasis

- Sepsis management
  - o Send cultures before starting antibiotics
  - o Within 3 hours → Start antibiotic (send cultures prior), bolus with 30cc/kg crystalloid if lactate >4
  - o Within 6 hours → Start pressors (norepinephrine recommended over dopamine, vasopressin added as secondary) if needed to maintain MAP, repeat lactate
  - o Activated protein C is no longer recommended (Never choose as an answer)
  - o Adrenal insufficiency in Septic Shock?
    - Generally do not do a stimulation test – if refractory shock and suspect adrenal insufficiency, you should empirically treat with hydrocortisone
  - o Glucose control in the ICU
    - Tight glucose control is associated with worse outcomes; shoot for <180

Vasoactive agents

- Dopamine
  - o Receptors:
    - Low dose: Dopamine receptors in kidney
    - Medium dose: Beta 1
    - High dose: Alpha

- Norepinephrine (Levophed)
  - o Receptors:
    - Alpha and some Beta 1

- Epinephrine
  - Receptors:
    - Alpha and Beta 1

- Phenylephrine
  - Receptors:
    - Purely alpha
  - Used in neurogenic shock from spinal cord injury

- Vasopressin
  - Receptors:
    - V1 receptor

- Dobutamine
  - Receptors:
    - Beta 1
  - Increases cardiac output
  - Can have vasodilatory effects

- Milrinone
  - Phosphodiesterase inhibitor
  - Increases cardiac output
  - Increases cAMP
  - Inotropic, Vasodilatory

Pulmonary Embolism (PE)

- Most common vital sign change?
  - Tachycardia, Tachypnea
  - Respiratory alkalosis

- Most common EKG findings with PE?
  - Sinus tachycardia
  - Classic S1Q3T3 finding is uncommon

- Diagnosis

- ○ CT Pulmonary Arteriogram is study of choice
- ○ Role of D-Dimer?
  - • Sensitive -- Good for ruling out PE. High false positive rate.
- • Treatment
  - ○ Anticoagulation – Heparin bolus followed by drip for goal PTT 60-90
  - ○ Indications for thrombolytics with PE?
    - • Hemodynamic instability
    - • Right heart strain on echocardiogram
  - ○ Pulmonary embolectomy (Trendelenburg Procedure)
    - • Uncommon
    - • Surgical option if there is a contraindication for lytics

Cardiovascular physiology

- • Central Venous Pressure (CVP) – surrogate for end diastolic right ventricular volume
- • Pulmonary Wedge Pressure (PWP) – surrogate for end diastolic left ventricular volume
- • Cardiac Output (CO)= Stroke volume x Heart Rate
- • Cardiac index (CI)= Cardiac Output/Body Surface Area
- • Swan Ganz Patterns – Less commonly used but good to know principles
  - ○ Hemorrhagic shock
  - ○ Low CO, High Systemic vascular resistance (SVR), Low filling pressures (CVP/PWP)
  - ○ Septic shock
    - • High CO (may be low in late septic shock), Low SVR, Low/ Normal filling pressures (CVP, PWP)
  - ○ Cardiogenic shock
    - • Low CO, High SVR, High filling pressures (CVP, PWP)

- Formulas you need to know
  - Oxygen Delivery = CO x [Hb x 02 Saturation x 1.34 + (Pa02 x 0.003)]
  - Oxygen Consumption = CO x (Arterial-Venous 02 difference)
  - Extraction Ratio = O2 Consumption/O2 Delivery
    - What decreases the Extraction Ratio?
      - Sepsis, cardiac failure, anemia/hypoxia, fever, seizure can affect extraction ratios

Anticoagulation Agents and reversal

- Coumadin – Inhibits Vit K dependent factors
  - Reversal:
    - FFP, Vit K
    - If emergent reversal needed → PCC
      - Less volume than FFP
      - Reversal is faster and more predictable than FFP

- Dabigatran (Pradaxa) – Direct Thrombin inhibitors
  - Reversal:
    - Dialysis
    - Praxbind – New monoclonal antibody against Pradaxa

- Apixaban (Eliquis), Rivaroxaban (Xarelto) – Factor Xa inhibitors
  - Reversal:
    - PCC will give partial reversal

Nutrition

- Metabolic Cart (Indirect Calorimetry)
  - Measures 02 Consumption and C02 production
  - Respiratory Quotient (RQ) = C02 production/02 consumption
  - RQ is useful to identify carbohydrate overfeeding in intubated patients, which results in higher C02 production and difficulty weaning from the ventilator.

- Fat 0.7
- Protein 0.8
- Carb 1.0

- Nitrogen balance
  - Requires 24-hour collection and measurement of urine Nitrogen
  - Nitrogen Balance = Protein intake /6.25 – (Urine nitrogen + 4)
    - Negative Nitrogen Balance = Catabolic State
    - Positive Nitrogen Balance = Anabolic State

- Caloric contents
  - Carb: 4 kcal/g
    - Should make up 75% of non-protein calories
    - Toxicity: CO_2 production, hyperglycemia, immunosuppressant
  - Dextrose: 3.4kCal/g
  - Lipids: 9 kcal/g
    - Should make up 25% of non-protein calories
    - Essential Fatty Acids
      - Linoleic acid
      - Alpha-Linolenic acid
    - Toxicity: pro-inflammatory (Omega 3 Fatty Acids are less inflammatory and immunogenic)
  - Protein: 4 kcal/g
    - 1-2 g/kg/day requirement

- Always prefer enteral nutrition over TPN if possible
  - Start enteral nutrition within 24-48hrs (after resuscitation/ stabilization)
  - If unable to tolerate enteral nutrition, start TPN at day 5-7

- Nutritional Deficiencies
  - Thiamine – Beri Beri
  - Folate – Macrocytic anemia
  - Vit D – Rickets
  - Vit C- Scurvy
  - Vit K – Coagulopathy
  - Zinc – rash, alopecia, vision changes
  - Copper – Microcytic anemia, pancytopenia, osteopenia
- Nutrition in pancreatitis patient
  - Classic teaching is to avoid gastric feeds and provide enteral nutrition with distal feeding access. More and more evidence showing gastric or small bowel enteral feeds generally acceptable. Trend is towards early enteral feeding.
- Immunonutrition – Contain Omega 3 fatty acids, Glutamine, Arginine
  - Associated with lower infectious complications

QUICK HITS

- Hemoptysis after Swan Ganz Balloon Inflation?
  - Ruptured pulmonary artery
  - Treatment: Angioembolization
- Tachyarrhythmia, Torsades de Pointes on EKG?
  - IV Magnesium
- No brainstem reflexes, fixed and dilated pupils, normotensive, normothermic. What's next to declare brain death?
  - Apnea Test
- Who should discuss organ donation with a brain dead patient's family?
  - The organ donation representative, not the physician.
- Hyperacute rejection of a transplanted organ is mediated by?
  - Antibodies

- Acute rejection of a transplanted organ is mediated by?
  - T-cells

- Cyclosporine/Tacrolimus mechanism of action?
  - Calcineurin inhibitor, blocks IL2

- Post Op Day 2 CABG patient with decreased chest tube output followed by PEA?
  - Cardiac Tamponade

  - Treatment: Cut wires and open chest in ICU

- Frequent IV Haldol doses for ETOH withdrawal followed by arrhythmia?
  - Prolonged QT

- Patient with positive UA with MAP of 60 and lactate of 4.5?
  - Septic Shock

- 5yo trauma patient with bradycardia during attempted intubation?
  - Atropine

- Post Op CABG patient with hypotension with CVP and wedge pressure of 20?
  - Cardiac Tamponade

- Critically ill patient in sudden drop in end tidal CO_2?
  - Decreased cardiac output or cardiac arrest

- Large volume paracentesis for ascites in a cirrhotic patient followed by oliguria and elevated Cr, Urine Na is less than 10?
  - Hepatorenal syndrome

  - Treatment: Albumin and vasopressin; transplant

16 FLUIDS AND ELECTROLYTES

- What is the percentage of total body water by weight in an adult? What percent of total body water is intracellular?
  - Body weight in Kg x 0.6 = L of water
  - 2/3rds is intracellular

- If 1/3rd of our total body water is extracellular, what percentage of that is intravascular?
  - ¼ is intravascular
  - ¾ is extravascular

- What is blood volume of 70 kg male?
  - 5 L
  - 7% by body weight
  - In pediatric it is 80 cc/kg

- What are our common maintenance fluids?
  - D5 ½ NS + 20 Meq of K
  - D5 ¼ NS in babies

- Resuscitative fluids?
  - Balanced crystalloid (LR or NS)
  - Colloids

- Electrolyte concentrations of NS and LR in 1L
  - NS = 154 mEq of Na and Cl
  - LR = 130 mEq sodium, 4 mEq potassium, 2.7 mEq calcium, 109 mEq chloride and 28 mEq of HCO3

- Maintenance fluids
  - 4, 2, 1 rule = hourly rate
  - 4 cc/kg for first 10 kg, 2 cc/kg for second 10, every 1 cc for every kg over 20 kg
  - Simplified version(for adults) = weight in kg + 40 = hourly rate of fluids

- How much sodium does a person need a day?
  - 1-2 mEq/kg
  - 70 kg person = 70-140 mEq/day

- How much potassium does a person need a day?
  - 0.5 -1 mEq/kg
  - 70 kg person = 35-70 mEq/day

- When to use D5 ½ NS?
  - Patients that are NPO
  - Protein sparing for fasting patients
  - D5 = 5% per liter = 50 Grams
  - 50 Grams x 3.4 kcal = 170 kcals per liter of D5 saline solution

- What fluid do you give to someone that has been copiously vomiting?
  - Resuscitative fluids (no D5), generally NS
  - 1 L at a time to see if they respond
  - ¼ of it stays intravascular

- How do colloids increase intravascular volume?
  - Oncotic pressure in vessel that draws fluids intravascular
  - Concern in sepsis/trauma/burns is with increased capillary permeability is colloid will leak out to interstitial space and draw fluid with it

- What colloids are available?
  - Albumin
  - Plasmanate
  - Hetastarch, Hespand
    - Side effects of coagulopathy
    - Negatively effects platelet function
    - Also can cause acute kidney injury

- What increases insensible losses?
  - Burns
  - Fevers
  - Ventilators
  - Open abdomen
  - Large open wounds

- What fluid do you replace with?
  - High NG tube output
    - Normal Saline
  - High volume bile leak (lose bicarb in bile)
    - LR or D5 solution with bicarb
  - Patient with diarrhea (lose K for colon)
    - LR or NS with K

- Patient 2 days s/p open procedure now hyponatremic what are possibilities?
  - Excess free water
  - SIADH
  - Pseudohyponatermia due to hyperglycemia or other high protein state
  - How to differentiate
  - Determine measured serum osmoles and calculated serum osmoles
  - Serum osmolality is calculated by looking at chemistry
    - Na, Glucose and BUN
    - $(2 \times Na) + Glucose/18 + BUN/2.8$
      - Simplified $(Na \times 2) + 10$
    - Compare to urine osmolality
    - If it is SIADH your serum osmolality will be less than urine (very concentrated urine)
    - If it is excess free water urine osmolality will be very low (trying to excrete excess water)

- o If it is excess free water how do you treat?
  - Fluid restriction
- o If it is SIADH?
  - Fluid restriction
  - Give NS (don't correct sodium too quickly, no more than 1 mEq/hour)
  - Vaptans (vasopressin antagonist)
  - Demeclocycline

- How to determine sodium deficit?
  - o Desired sodium – actual sodium x TBW = Sodium deficit in mEq

- Primary causes of hypernatremia?
  - o Iatrogenic
  - o Diabetes insipidus
  - o Pt with head injury and urine output increases to 700 cc/hr and now hypernatremic how to confirm its DI?
    - Compare serum osmolality to urine osmolality
    - Serum osmolality will be high and urine will be low in DI
  - o How to treat DI?
    - Desmopressin (DDAVP)
  - o How to calculate free water deficit
    - (Actual Na – Desired Na)/ Desired Na x TBW = Volume in liters

- What is hypophosphatemia associated with?
  - o Refeeding syndrome due to P04 shift extracellular to intracellular
  - o Can lead to failure to wean from ventilator

- How do you manage patient with hyperkalemia?
  - o Likely renal failure, could be medication induced
  - o EKG looking for peaked T waves

- o Treatment
  - Give calcium to stabilize myocardium
  - NaHCO3
  - Glucose with IV Insulin
  - Lasix
  - Kayexalate
  - Albuterol
  - Emergent Dialysis

- How to treat hypokalemia?
  - o Causes – Iatrogenic such as over diuresis
  - o 40 mEq of K should increase total K 0.4

- Hypocalcemia symptoms
  - o Weakness
  - o Perioral Tingling
  - o Chovstek's sign – tap on facial nerve and get perioral twitching
  - o Trousseau's sign – Carpal pedal spasm with blood pressure cuff

- Treatment of hypocalcemia?
  - o IV Calcium
  - o Vit D and Mg

- If hypocalcemia patient has low serum albumin, how do we correct serum calcium?
  - o Normal Albumin = 4
  - o Every point below 4 add 0.8 to calcium level
  - o If Albumin = 2, add 1.6 to serum calcium level

- What are main causes of hypercalcemia?
  - o MC cause of hypercalcemia in outpatient = hyperparathyroidism
  - o MC cause of hypercalcemia in an inpatient = malignancy

- Symptoms of hypercalcemia?
  - Stones, bones, groans, and psychiatric overtones
  - Kidney stones, bone pain, abdominal pain, and psychosis

- Treatment of hypercalcemia?
  - Crystalloid resuscitation
  - Loop diuretic second line
  - Bisphosphonates are helpful for hypercalcemia due to cancer
  - Calcitonin
  - Glucocorticoids
  - Dialysis

- Most important parts of ABG?
  - pCO2, Bicarb, Base Excess/Base Deficit

- Normal values of ABG (to remember for exam)
  - pCO2 = 40
  - pH = 7.4
  - Bicarb = 24

- A change in pCO2 what change in pH would you expect?
  - $0.8 \times \Delta CO2 = \Delta pH$ for acute changes
  - pH change by .1 for every 12 point change in CO2

- Dr. Matthew Martin Tips When Looking at ABG
  - Looks at CO2 first
    - If high writes resp acidosis. If low, writes resp alkalosis
  - Then looks at bicarb
    - If high, writes metabolic alkalosis. If low, writes metabolic acidosis
  - Then he looks at pH and their history to put it all together

- Metabolic acidosis
  - Start with calculating anion gap
  - (Na + K) – (Cl + HCO3)
  - Gap Acidosis = MUDPILES
  - Non-Anion Gap = Ileal conduit, Fistulas, Hyperchloremic (Too much NaCL), Renal Tubular Acidosis, Diarrhea, Acetazolamide

- Metabolic alkalosis
  - NG suction – Hyperchloremic, hypokalemic metabolic alkalosis
  - Contraction alkalosis from over diuresis
    - Give chloride back is most important

Electrolyte Abnormality	Signs and Symptoms	Basic Treatments
Hypernatremia (DI)	↑ urine output ± head injury, ↑ serum osm, ↓urine osm	Desmopressin (DDAVP)
Hyponatremia (excess free water)	↓↓ urine osm	Fluid restriction
Hyponatremia (SIADH)	Serum osm < urine osm	Fluid restrict, NS, Vaptans, demeclocycline
Hyperkalemia	Peaked T waves on EKG, arrhythmias	Calcium to stabilize myocardium Glucose + IV insulin, albuterol Lasix, sodium bicarbonate Kayexalate Emergent Dialysis
Hypokalemia	Fatigue, weakness, muscle cramps or twitches	Potassium supplementation Magnesium
Hypophosphatemia (refeeding syndrome)	Fatigue, weakness, arrhythmias, confusion, seizures	Low and slow nutritional supplementation to start
Hypercalcemia	Stones, bones, groans, psychiatric overtones	Crystalloid resuscitation Loop diuretics (2nd line) Bisphosphonates (cancer) Calcitonin, glucocorticoids Dialysis
Hypocalcemia	Perioral tingling, weakness Chvostek's sign Trousseau's sign	IV calcium Magnesium Vitamin D

Table 1: Common Electrolyte Abnormalities and Treatment

Acid Base Practice Problems

- Patient undergoes surgery and has 3L NG Suction, postop ABG shows 7.55, pCO2= 52, HCO3 = 40
  - What is his primary disorder?
    - He is alkalotic with a metabolic alkalosis (HCO3 of 40)
    - Respiratory acidosis is compensatory
    - Primary metabolic alkalosis with respiratory compensation

- Patient who is admitted in a coma, pCO2 = 16, HCO3 = 5, pH = 7.1
  - Metabolic acidosis with a respiratory compensation
  - Respiratory alkalosis is compensatory as overall disorder is acidotic

- Climber climbing a mountain, he is at 5000 meters, what is his going to happen to his pCO2 and his pH?
  - pCO2 will go down and pH will go up
  - Respiratory alkalosis

- Patient whose pH is 7.5, PCO2 = 50, HCO3 is 35
  - Primarily metabolic alkalosis with respiratory compensation

Quick Hits

- Cation that determines serum osmolarity
  - Na

- Primary intracellular cation
  - K

- Sepsis resuscitation bolus amount cc/kg
  - 30cc/kg

- Pediatric patient who needs bolus
  - 20 cc/kg
  - Blood products = 10 cc/kg

- Pt with K of 6.5 and peaked T waves on EKG, what medication do you give first
  - Calcium gluconate

- Pt on liver transplant list, who was started on a "water pill" by his PCP, now has K of 2.5
  - Lasix

- Pt on liver transplant list, who was started on a "water pill" by his PCP, now his K is 5.5
  - Spironolactone

- Pt came in hyponatremic getting 3% NS, and now they develop spastic quadriplegia
  - Central pontine myelinolysis

- Pt is hyponatremic, they are on free water restriction, still hyponatremic
  - Can give vaptans (acts on V2 receptor in the kidney) or demeclocycline
  - Or hypertonic saline

- Baby with pyloric stenosis who has been having emesis for 1 week
  - Hypochloremic, hypokalemic, metabolic acidosis
  - Paradoxical aciduria

- Effect of acidosis on oxygen-hemoglobin disassociation curve
  - Right shift – oxygen will unload easier

- Surgical patient gets hextend and is now bleeding in OR, what coagulation disorder do they have
  - Platelet dysfunction

- Pt with marked metabolic alkalosis, now has decreased respiratory drive, what drug could you give
  - Acetazolamide

- Pt with high NG output, or vomiting
  - Hypochloremic, metabolic alkaloses

- Pt with diarrhea
  - Hypokalemic metabolic acidosis

- Mountain climber
  - Respiratory alkalosis

- POD 2 after whipple is now somnolent with pinpoint pupils
  - Respiratory acidosis, due to overdose on narcotics

- Ileal conduit and high output
  - Metabolic acidosis, non-gap

17 HERNIAS

Basic Principles

Underlying principle of good hernia repair = Tension free
Most common cause for recurrent hernia = wound infection
Rank as cause of SBO = 2nd to adhesion (worldwide = 1st)

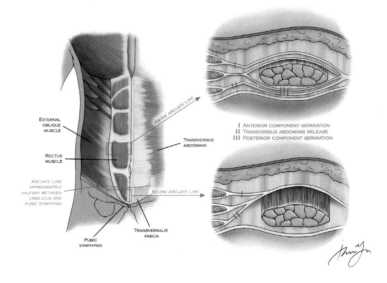

Figure 1 - Abdominal Wall Anatomy

Abdominal Wall Anatomy

- Layers of abdominal wall just off midline:
  - Skin
  - Subcutaneous Fat/Camper's Fascia
  - Scarpa's Fascia
  - Anterior Rectus Sheath
  - Rectus Muscle
  - Posterior Rectus Sheath
  - Preperitoneal Fat
  - Peritoneum

- Layers of abdominal wall lateral to rectus:
  - Skin
  - Subcutaneous Fat/Camper's Fascia

- o Scarpa's Fascia
- o External Oblique
- o Internal Oblique
- o Transversus Abdominis
- o Transversalis Fascia
- o Preperitoneal Fat
- o Peritoneum

- Where does rectus sheath end?
  - o Arcuate line (third of distance between umbilicus and pubis symphysis)

- Bloody supply to the rectus?
  - o Inferior and Superior Epigastrics

- Hesselbach's Triangle Anatomy
  - o Medial Border – Rectus
  - o Inferior Border – Inguinal Ligament
  - o Lateral Border – Epigastrics
  - o Hernia in Hesselbach's triangle = Direct Hernia

- What is the inguinal ligament?
  - o Extension of the external oblique fascia

- What are the embryological structures that are at or go through umbilicus?
  - o Omphalomesenteric duct (Vitelline duct) → Becomes Meckel's Diverticulum
  - o Median umbilical ligament → urachus
  - o Medial umbilical ligaments → obliterated umbilical arteries
  - o Round ligament of the liver (ligamentum teres) → obliterated umbilical vein

- When does the midgut herniate? And what does it return?
  - o Herniates at 6 weeks
  - o Returns at 10 weeks

- Abdominal wall defect in Omphalocele? Gastroschisis?
  - o Omphalocele → Through the umbilical stalk
  - o Gastroschisis → Inferior/Right of the umbilicus

Umbilical Hernias

- Usually congenital

- Usual contents → preperitoneal fat

- Repair options?
  - o Open vs. Laparoscopic
  - o Primary repair → <1cm and pediatric patients

- 2 yo with umbilical hernia
  - o Wait until 5yo to see if it will close and then repair
  - o Fix before going to school

Inguinal Hernias

- What defines indirect/direct hernia?
  - o Indirect is lateral to inferior epigastrics
  - o Direct is medial to inferior epigastrics

- Etiology of indirect?
  - o Congenital - Patent processus vaginalis

- Etiology of direct?
  - o Acquired - Weakness in floor of inguinal canal

- Risk factors for direct?
  - o Obesity, smoking, poor nutrition, ascites, anything with increased abdominal pressure

- Contents of spermatic cord?
  - o Cremasteric muscles, testicular artery, vas deferens, pampiniform plexus, ilioinguinal nerve, genital branch of genitofemoral nerve

- What forms the cremaster muscles?
  - o Extension of the internal oblique muscle fibers

- What are the key nerves in open inguinal hernia repair?
  - Ilioinguinal
  - Genital branch of genitofemoral
  - Iliohypogastric
  - MC injured → Ilioinguinal (when opening external oblique)

- MC injured nerve in laparoscopic hernia repair
  - Lateral femoral cutaneous
    - Occurs from improperly placed tack laterally

- Bassini
  - Conjoint tendon (transversalis + internal oblique) to inguinal ligament

- Shouldice
  - Same as bassini in multiple (4) layers

- Lichtenstein repair
  - Repair with mesh, sew inguinal ligament to conjoined/ transversalis

- Plug and patch
  - Plug goes into internal repair and then Lichtenstein on top

- Pediatric repair basics?
  - High ligation of sac

- Laparoscopic hernia repair
  - Total Extra-Peritoneal Repair (TEP) and Trans-Abdominal Pre-Peritoneal Repair (TAPP)
  - Repair covers internal, direct, and femoral spaces
  - Main structure of fixation in laparoscopic repair?
    - Cooper's ligament
  - What and where is the triangle of doom?
    - Contains Iliac vessels, medial with apex at iliopubic tract and bounded by vas deferens medially and spermatic vessels laterally

o What and where is the triangle of pain?

- Contains Nerve structures, lateral to spermatic vessels below iliopubic tract

Femoral Hernias

- Who is at highest risk for femoral hernias?
  o Females and elderly

- Where is the defect?
  o Below the inguinal ligament, medial to the femoral vein

- How do you repair it open?
  o McVay (Cooper's) Repair

  - Open inguinal floor, close femoral space by suturing Conjoint tendon to Cooper's Ligament

Incarceration vs. Strangulation

- What are the signs of symptoms?
  o Obstructive, non-reducible hernia, skin changes, severe tenderness and pain

- Open approach and needed bowel resection. How do you repair?
  o Biologic mesh or tissue repair

Ventral/Incisional Hernias

- Risks Factors for incisional hernia?
  o Wound infection, obesity, COPD, smoking

  o GET THEM TO STOP SMOKING prior to elective repair

  o Where can you place the mesh?

  - Underlay, inlay, onlay

  - Highest recurrence in inlay mesh

  - Choose macroporous mesh

  - Biologic mesh if contamination

  o How to manage large ventral hernia if you cannot obtain

primary closure?

- Component separation -- There are several types/ variations. A common board question regards which layer is incised (See Image).
  - Anterior Component Separation (incise external oblique)
  - Transversus Abdominis Repair (incise transversus abdominis)
  - Posterior Component Separation (incise posterior rectus sheath)
- o Optimal suture closer method?
  - 5-7mm bites with absorbable suture

Quick Hits

- Junction of semilunaris and arcuate line?
  - o Spigelian hernia → intramuscular hernia

- Appendix in inguinal hernia sac?
  - o Amyand hernia, primary repair in appendicitis

- Meckel's diverticulum in inguinal hernia?
  - o Littre's hernia

- Both indirect and direct hernia?
  - o Pantaloon hernia

- Sliding hernia?
  - o Retroperitoneal structure makes up a portion of the sac
  - o Do not open sac with a sliding hernia

- Richter's hernia
  - o Part of the wall of the bowel is present in the hernia sac
  - o Strangulation without obstruction

- Doing inguinal hernia repair and skeletonized cord and can't find hernia?
  - o Need to open floor and look for femoral hernia

- Child's C cirrhotic with massive ascites and umbilical hernia with intermittent obstructive symptoms?
  - TIPS first to control ascites before considering repair

- Laparoscopic inguinal hernia repair and tack mesh to cooper's ligament and get large arterial bleeding?
  - Corona mortis (branch between obturator and external iliac artery)

- Placing suture during open inguinal hernia repair and get sudden bleeding?
  - Femoral vein injury, pull suture out and hold pressure

- Groin pain/significant medial thigh pain with internal rotation of the hip?
  - Obturator hernia
  - Obturator sign/Howship Romberg sign

- One-month s/p open inguinal hernia repair with prolene mesh and now have wound infection with purulent fluid around mesh?
  - Mesh explantation

- Inguinal hernia repair and can't reduce sac
  - Ligate proximal portion that will reduce into abdominal cavity
  - Keep distal portion open to reduce chances of hydrocele

18 THORACIC

High Yield Anatomy

- How many lobes on the right vs left?
  - 3 vs 2 anatomic lobes

- What is a good way to remember the lymph node stations?
  - Single digits are mediastinal vs double digits are hilar

- What is the full course of the thoracic duct?
  - Cisterna chyli (L2) → crosses at T5 from right to left → empties into junction of L internal jugular and subclavian veins

  - What is the final destination of the azygous?

    - Superior vena cava

> Where do you find the duck (thoracic duct)?
> Between the two goose – azyGOOSE vein and esophaGOOSE

- Where do the nerves run in relation to the hilum of the lung?
  - Phrenic nerve is anterior

  - oVagus nerve runs posterior

> Think alphabetical order: A (anterior) before P (posterior)
> P (phrenic) → anterior comes before V (vagus) → posterior

- What are the anatomic boundaries of the mediastinum?
  - Sternum anteriorly, vertebrae posteriorly, pleurae laterally, thoracic inlet superiorly, diaphragm inferiorly

- What are the types of pneumocytes and their function?
  - Type 1 = gas exchange

  - Type 2 = makes surfactant (phosphatidylcholine is the primary component)

- What are the pores of Kahn?
  - Pores in alveoli that enable direct air exchange

Space of Disse is the hepatic analog: hepatocytes interact directly with the sinusoids

Functional Definitions

- o Pulmonary Function Tests
  - What is the pre-op workup of a patient you are considering for lobectomy?
    - Predicted forced expiratory volume FEV1 > 0.8 (80%)
      - o If close → V/Q scan will show contribution of the diseased lung
    - FEV1 is the best predictor of post op complications. What else is predictive of increased perioperative risk?
      - o Diffusion capacity of the lung for CO_2 or DLCO < 10 mL/min/mm (40% predicted)
- o What is Light's criteria?
  - Characterize pleural fluid as exudate vs transudate
    - Pleural:serum protein ratio > 0.5
    - Pleural:serum LDH ratio > 0.6
    - Pleural LDH > 2/3 of normal serum LDH

Pleural disease

- Pleural effusion and Empyema
  - o What causes these?
    - Increased permeability of the pleura and capillaries (sepsis, malignancy, pancreatitis)
    - Increased hydrostatic pressure (CHF, CKD)
    - Hypoalbuminemia (cirrhosis, nephrotic syndrome, malnutrition)
  - o What type of imaging should you get and what would you see?
    - CXR = blunting of costophrenic angle, visible effusion if > 300 mL, fluid in fissures

- US = fluid in the pleural space with loss of inspiratory sliding
- CT chest = simple effusion will be homogeneous, most are posterior and inferior vs an empyema would be a loculated, heterogeneous collection
  - o Treatment?
    - Pleural effusion → conservative management, treat underlying cause, unless symptomatic then drain
    - Empyema → decortication

- How do you manage a retained hemothorax?
  - o Chest tube → VATS or thoracotomy for washout

- Chylothorax
  - o How do you diagnose it?
    - Milky white fluid
    - > 110 mg/dL triglycerides with lymphocyte predominance
    - Sudan red stains fat and will be positive
  - o What are the most common etiologies?
    - 50% are due to malignancy (lymphoma)
    - What causes the other 50%?
      - Trauma or iatrogenic
      - When do symptoms begin after iatrogenic injury?
        - o After initiation of oral intake
  - o What is the management?
    - First-line is conservative management with low fat, medium-chain fatty acid diet (no long-chain FAs) or bowel rest with TPN if high-volume or persistent leak on the oral diet, chest tube if necessary, +/- octreotide
    - If fails or due to traumatic injury → ligation of thoracic duct in low right mediastinum vs talc pleurodesis and possible chemoradiation for malignancy

- 18-year-old basketball player, occasionally uses marijuana, suddenly felt chest pain with inspiration while watching TV.

What does he likely have?

○ Spontaneous pneumothorax due to apical subpleural blebs

○ What is the difference between primary and secondary PTX?

- Secondary is due to an underlying medical condition. Examples?

  - COPD most common, asthma, CF, infection, malignancy, connective tissue disease, congenital cysts, etc.

○ ED confirmed PTX on CXR and intern goes down to see. At this point he looks anxious, working a bit to breathe, HR 120, RR 30, BP 90/50, with a prominent neck vein. What does he have?

- Tension pneumothorax - if the intern isn't too far into surgical residency, he/she probably took a stethoscope and heard an absence of breath sounds on the affected side

- What is the first step in managing this?

  - Needle decompression

  - How would you do that?

    ○ Insert a needle, angiocaths are readily available, into the second intercostal space at a 90-degree angle to the chest, just over the third rib.

  - In reality, we would place a chest tube which would be just as quick

○ Back to non-tension PTX. How do you manage these?

- For clinically stable with small PTX → observe

- For clinically stable with large (> 3 cm) → pigtail catheter or chest tube

- For unstable and large → chest tube

- When do you operate?

  - Persistent air leak (> 4 days) → VATS with pleurodesis

  - After second recurrence of spontaneous/primary → blebectomy

  - High-risk profession after first occurrence (scuba diver, pilot)

> Spontaneous pneumothorax in the OR, don't see blebs.
> What do you do? Apical wedge resection

- How do you perform a pleurodesis?
  - Can do mechanical with scratch pad, bovie, etc.
  - Chemical = doxycycline, bleomycin, talc
  - Pleurectomy
  - Indwelling intrapleural catheter
  - Goal is to abut the visceral and parietal pleura by causing an inflammatory reaction that scars them together

Mediastinal disease

- o 60-year-old alcoholic went on a binge and had massive, forceful emesis. Comes to the ED with chest pain, fever, tachycardia. CXR unremarkable. Next step?
  - Worried about esophageal perforation so gastrografin swallow; also need to see extent of mediastinitis → CT neck/chest with PO and IV contrast
  - Acute mediastinitis usually due to acute perforation of esophagus or trachea and can lead to descending necrotizing infection → sepsis
    - Can also be caused by oropharyngeal infections (Ludwig angina)
  - Chronic mediastinitis usually manifests as fibrosis
  - How do you manage acute mediastinal infection?
    - Source control, antibiotics → sternal debridement if postop sternotomy is the etiology, cervical drain if cervical infection, VATS to drain mediastinum into pleural space if lower mediastinal infection
- o Mediastinal tumors
  - Most common cause of mediastinal adenopathy?
    - Lymphoma
  - Most common overall type of mediastinal tumor in adults and children?

- Neurogenic (posterior mediastinum)
- Most common site of mediastinal tumor?
  - Anterior = terrible Ts → thymoma, teratoma, thyroid (ectopic), (terrible) lymphoma
  - What else do you need to check in a male who presents with a mediastinal mass?
    - ○ Scrotum (germ cell tumor)
- Most common germ cell tumor?
  - Teratoma
  - And where is that located?
    - ○ Anterior mediastinum
- Thymomas and myasthenia gravis
  - 50% of thymomas are malignant
  - 50% are symptomatic
  - 50% have myasthenia
  - 10% of patients with myasthenia have a thymoma
  - 80% of myasthenia patients will improve with thymectomy
- ○ Superior vena cava syndrome
  - Causes?
    - Malignancy most common (60%) → small cell lung cancer most common, then lymphoma
    - Nonmalignant = fibrosing mediastinits, substernal thyroid goiter, sarcoid, etc., secondary to indwelling intravascular devices
  - How do they present?
    - Venous obstructive symptoms with dilation of head and neck veins and facial, neck, or arm swelling; can get laryngeal and tracheobronchial compression
    - Fullness in the head when bending over
    - Can be associated with Horner syndrome if due to a pancoast tumor = ptosis, miosis, anhidrosis

- Diagnosis: CXR, CT with contrast, +/- venography
- Treatment = position patient to reduce edema, steroids, +/- anticoagulation, emergent radiation if very symptomatic, treat underlying cause

Lung Masses

○ What are the screening recommendations?

- Annual low-dose CT for 3 years in 55-80-year-old current or former smokers with > 30 pack-year history or quit within the past 15 years

○ Is lung cancer still the #1 cause of cancer-related death in the US?

- Yes
- Strongest prognostic indicator?
    - Nodal involvement
- Most common site of metastases?
    - Brain (also goes to supraclavicular nodes, contralateral lung, bone, liver, adrenal)

○ Solitary pulmonary nodule

- What is the workup?
    - Must ask 2 questions:
        ○ Is it a benign calcification or stable for 2 years? → no further work up
        ○ Is the surgical risk acceptable? If no, consider biopsy for diagnosis and radiation for palliation if necessary
        ○ If growing over 2 years but acceptable surgical risk, consider clinical probability of cancer
            - Low → serial CT at 3, 6, 12, 24 months
            - Intermediate → PET/CT, transthoracic or bronchoscopic biopsy
            - High → VATS biopsy with frozen section and then lobectomy if malignant

o Lung cancer

- What is the most common type of lung cancer?

  - Non-small cell (80%)

  - Squamous and small cell are more central versus adenocarcinoma is peripheral

- There are some paraneoplastic syndromes associated with lung cancer, what are they?

  - Squamous cell = PTH-related peptide causing hypercalcemia

  - Small cell = ACTH (most common paraneoplastic syndrome) and ADH secretion

- When do you perform mediastinoscopy?

  - Centrally located tumors or suspicious adenopathy

  - Positive mediastinal nodes = unresectable tumor

> Mediastinal nodes are single digits.

- Which nodes are not assessed?

  - o Aortopulmonary

  - o Need to perform Chamberlain procedure = anterior thoracotomy or parasternal mediastinotomy through L 2nd rib cartilage

- What is the TNM staging?

  - T stages

    - o T1 < 3 cm

    - o T2 3-5 cm

    - o T3 5-7 or invading chest wall or pericardium

    - o T4 > 7 cm or invading mediastinum, etc.

  - N stages

    - o N3 = supraclavicular or cervical LN

- Metastases
  - o Hematogenous spread to brain, adrenals, contralateral lung, bone
  - o MRI brain for neurologic complaints, Stage III/IV or small cell and Pancoast tumors
- What is the treatment?
  - Stage I and II = resection or definitive radiation if not a surgical candidate
  - Locally advanced Stage III can be resected after neoadjuvant chemoXRT
  - Stage IIIb with T4 tumor or N3 lymph nodes require chemoradiation
  - Stage IV usually palliative resection or radiation
  - When can you do VATS versus open resection?
    - o Tumor < 5 cm, peripheral, no regional lymphadenopathy or local invasion
- What are the surveillance recommendations?
  - Stage I/II: H&P with CT chest every 6 months for 3 years → annual H&P with noncontrast CT chest
  - Stage III/IV: H&P with CT chest every 3-6 months for 3 years → H&P with CT chest every 6 months → annual

Trauma

- o What volume of blood from a chest tube indicates need for OR?
  - 1500 mL initially or 200-300 mL/h for 2-4 hours
- o What are the indications for a resuscitative thoracotomy?
  - Penetrating injury with < 15 min CPR
  - Penetrating extrathoracic injury with exsanguination and < 5 minutes CPR
  - Blunt trauma losing vital signs en route or witnessed in ED with < 10 min CPR

- o What are the steps in a resuscitative thoracotomy?
  - Nasogastric or orogastric tube to help identify esophagus
  - Double lumen intubation to deflate lung on side of injury
  - Anterolateral incision to enter chest → rib spreader → pericardiotomy and control cardiac injury, cross clamp aorta, cardiac massage

Quick Hits

- Massive bleeding in patient with tracheostomy. What is it? Management?
  - o Tracheoinnominate fistula
  - o Temporizing measures: inflate cuff, anterior pressure of finger through trach opening
  - o Place trach hole and rush to OR for median sternotomy and ligation and resection of innominate artery

| Do not pick reconstruction of the artery, it will blow out. |

- o How do you prevent this fistula?
  - Place trach between 2nd and 3rd tracheal ring

- Do pericardial cysts have to be resected?
  - o No if asymptomatic, find them at the right costobronchial angle

- Do bronchiogenic cysts have to be resected?
  - o Yes, find them posterior to carina

- Most common benign/malignant tumor in adults?
  - o Benign: Hamartoma
    - Popcorn lesion +/- calcifications
    - No treatment → repeat CT in 6 months to confirm diagnosis
  - o Malignant: squamous cell carcinoma

- Most common tumors in children?
  - o Benign: Hemangioma
  - o Malignant: Carcinoid

- What type of lung cancer mimics pneumonia?
  - o Bronchoalveolar cancer and it grows along the alveolar walls, usually multifocal

19 PEDIATRIC SURGERY

Trauma

- #1 cause of death in children
- What is the best indicator of shock in pediatric patients?
  - Tachycardia
  - Children look well until they decompensate quickly

> Tachycardia by age group (general rule of thumb):
> Neonate = > 150 beats per minute
> Age 1 - 6 = > 120 bpm
> Age 6 – 12 = > 110 bpm
> Age 13+ = same as adult

- What are the targets for fluid resuscitation?
  - Crystalloid = 20 mL/kg
  - Blood = 10 mL/kg (give after 2 fluid boluses in hypotensive)
  - UOP = 2-3 mL/kg/hr in neonate/infant, 1 mL/kg/hr in toddlers and older
  - MIVF = 4 mL/kg/hr for 1st 10 kg → 2 for 2nd 10 → 1 for the rest
- How do you choose ETT in children < 10 years old?
  - Uncuffed tube for neonates only
  - Size = , size of pinkie, or Breslow tape

Emesis

Important to know age group for most common presentations and bilious vs non-bilious

- What is the differential by age?
  - Neonates
    - Nonsurgical: infectious, allergy, metabolic disorder
    - Surgical: GERD, pyloric stenosis, intestinal obstruction, atresia

- o Infants/toddlers
  - Nonsurgical: infectious, neurologic/psychologic, gastroparesis
  - Surgical: intussusception
- o Adolescents
  - Nonsurgical: functional disorder, IBD, psychologic
  - Surgical: appendicitis
- What is the differential for non-bilious emesis?
  - o Pyloric stenosis
    - Buzz words: projectile vomiting, olive mass
    - Metabolic disturbance: HYPOchloremic, HYPOkalemic, metabolic alkalosis + paradoxic aciduria
    - Diagnosis = ultrasound → pylorus > 4 mm thick and > 14 mm long

> **PI**loric stenosis (pi = 3.14): > 3mm thick and > 14 mm long

- Treatment = RESUSCITATE first with normal saline → dextrose containing MIVF → OR for pyloromyotomy

> Do not resuscitate with lactated Ringer's, which contains potassium, until metabolic disturbance is resolved.

  - o What are the features of tracheoesophageal fistula?
    - Five types
      - Type C most common with blind ending esophageal atresia and distal TE fistula
      - Type A is the next most common and is the only one without a TE fistula, just esophageal atresia
- Diagnosis = AXR (Type C will have gas + distended stomach vs Type A will be gasless)
  - Important in diagnostic workup- check for VACTERL
  - What are the VACTERL syndrome components?

- o Vertebral anomalies → sacral US
- o Anorectal- imperforate anus → rectal exam
  - Presentation: meconium in urine or vagina from fistula if high or to perineal skin if low
  - Treatment = above levators need colostomy first, below levators straight to posterior sagittal anoplasty + postop anal dilation
- o Cardiac → echocardiogram
- o **TE** fistula
- o Renal → US
- o **L**imb anomalies

- Treatment = resuscitate with Replogle tube (double-lumen tube to suction saliva and keep esophagus patent) → G-tube + primary repair (right extrapleural thoracotomy)

- Common complications: similar to esophagectomy → GERD, leak, stricture, fistula

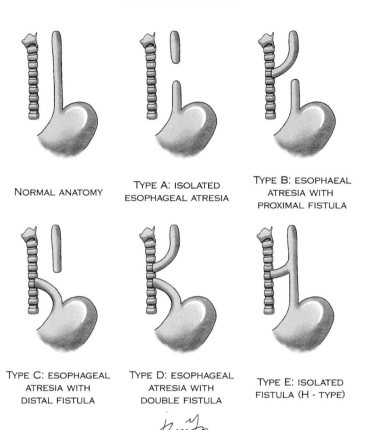

Figure 1 – Types of trachea-esophageal fistulae

○ Intussusception (will be bilious if obstructed)

- Buzz words: currant jelly stools, target sign on imaging
- Underlying etiology: #1 inflamed Peyer's patches after viral illness, #2 lymphoma, #3 Meckel's diverticulum

Intussusception in adults are commonly caused by a malignant lead point → OR, no air contrast enema

- Diagnosis = US
- Treatment = air-contrast enema
  - What if it recurs?
    - o 15% recur, repeat air-contrast enema
  - When do you operate?
    - o If unable to reduce with enema, peritonitis, obstruction

 After successful reduction with enema → observe for 4 hours, PO challenge, discharge

- What is the differential for bilious emesis?
  - o Malrotation with midgut volvulus (malrotation on its own is asymptomatic)
    - Malrotation etiology = failure of normal 270-degree rotation during intestinal development
    - Volvulus caused by Ladd's bands (adhesions from right retroperitoneum)
      - If child with malrotation is going to develop volvulus, majority present by 1 year old
    - Diagnosis = always #1 on differential in pediatric bilious emesis → emergent upper GI to rule it out (duodenum doesn't cross midline)
    - Associations: CDH in 20%, omphalocele
    - Treatment = resect Ladd's bands and counterclockwise detorsion to place small intestine on right and large intestine on left + appendectomy (to avoid future diagnostic uncertainty)

 Turn back time: counterclockwise detorsion

  - o Duodenal atresia
    - Buzz words: double-bubble sign on X-ray (image search this)

- #1 cause of duodenal obstruction in neonates
- What are some associations?
  - Polyhydramnios (not swallowing the amniotic fluid)
  - Cardiac, renal, GI anomalies
  - Down's syndrome in 20%
- Diagnosis = AXR + UGI
- Treatment = resuscitate → reconnect to duodenum or jejunum
- Other intestinal atresias are due to intrauterine vascular accidents – most commonly in jejunum and can be multiple

> Duodenal atresia is caused by failure of recanalization

○ Meconium ileus
- Presentation: no meconium passed in first 24 hours
- Diagnosis = AXR shows dilated small bowel without air-fluid level + sweat chloride test
- Association: 10% of cystic fibrosis patients
- Treatment = Gastrogafin enema or N-acetylcysteine (NAC) enema
  - When should you operate?
    ○ Perforation, ostomy creation for antegrade NAC enemas
- What's another disease that doesn't pass meconium in first 24 hours?
  - Hirschsprung's disease
    ○ #1 cause of colonic obstruction in infants, 2-3 years old will have chronic constipation
    ○ Presentation: distention +/- colitis
    ○ Diagnosis = suction rectal biopsy → absent ganglion cells in myenteric plexus (due to failure to progress caudad)

- o Treatment = resect rectum and colon until ganglion cells present → can reconnect colon to anus later

  - • If colitis (foul smelling diarrhea, sepsis) → rectal irrigation +/- emergency colectomy

Bloody stools

- o Intussusception - remember currant jelly stools

- o How does necrotizing enterocolitis present?

  - • Bloody stools after 1st feeding, premature baby, abdominal distension, septic

  - • Diagnosis = AXR → pneumatosis (not an indication for surgery alone), free air, portal venous gas (portends poor prognosis) + serial lateral decubitus films to monitor for perforation

  - • Treatment = resuscitate, NPO, Abx, TPN, orogastric tube

    - • When to operate?

      - o Pneumoperitoneum, peritonitis, clinical deterioration, abdominal wall erythema

    - • Barium enema prior to taking down ostomies down the road to rule out stenotic distal obstruction

- o What is a Meckel's diverticulum?

  - • Due to persistent vitelline (omphalomesenteric) duct

  - • Presentation: painless lower GI bleed most commonly

  - • What is the rule of 2s?

    - • 2 inches long

    - • 2 cm diameter

    - • < 2 years old

    - • 2:1 male to female predominance

    - • 2 feet from ileocecal valve

    - • 2% of the population

    - • 2% symptomatic

    - • 2 types of tissue- pancreatic and gastric

- o Gastric most likely to be symptomatic
- • 2 presentations – diverticulitis and bleeding
- • Diagnosis = Meckel's scan for operative preparation (will only pick up gastric mucosa)
- • Treatment = resection of diverticulum + segmental resection if involving base or >1/3 size of bowel or diverticulitis

Abdominal Wall Defects

	Gastroschisis	Omphalocele
Etiology	In utero rupture of umbilical vein	Failure of embryonal development
Sac	No	Yes - can contain other organs
Location	Right of midline	Midline
Associations	Intestinal atresia (most common), malrotation	–
Diagnosis	Obstetric ultrasound	Obstetric ultrasound
Treatment	Moist wrap + resuscitation + TPN/NPO → replace bowel and primary closure of silastic mesh silo	Same as gastroschisis
Prognosis	Better than omphalocele	Worse than gastroschisis

Table 1 – Features of gastroschisis versus omphalocele

O in omphalocele: looks like a complete sac (covered by peritoneum), looks like a belly button (midline)

- o When do you repair a pediatric umbilical hernia?
  - • If it hasn't closed by 5 years of age
- o What is the etiology of inguinal hernias?
  - • Due to persistent processus vaginalis
  - • Treatment = elective high ligation of sac, OR within 72 hours of reduction if incarcerated
    - • Explore contralateral side if left-sided, female, or < 1 year old

In adults, hernias are typically repaired with resection of the hernia sac.

- Hydrocele similar but no sac extending into internal ring
  - Communicating vs noncommunicating
    - ○ Noncommunicating usually resolve by 1 year
    - ○ Communicating wax and wane
  - Treatment = surgery at 1 year old if not resolved or communicating → resect hydrocele and ligate processus vaginalis
- ○ What are the features of undescended testicles?
  - Associations: risk of testicular CA even after orchiopexy, seminoma, chromosomal disorder if undescended bilaterally
  - Treatment = orchiopexy (can divide spermatic vessels because of vas deferens collateral)

Abdominal Masses

- ○ How do neuroblastomas present?
  - Usually asymptomatic, can have HTN, diarrhea, raccoon eyes from orbital metastases, or unsteady gait
    - Most commonly adrenal, but can be anywhere along sympathetic chain
    - Most commonly < 2 years old with best prognosis if < 1 year old
    - Rarely metastasizes
  - Diagnosis = catecholamines, metanephrines VMA, HVA, AXR showing stippled calcifications, CT showing renal displacement (vs Wilms replaces parenchyma)
    - High risk/worse prognosis: neuron-specific enolase, LDH, HVA, diploid tumor, N-myc amplification

Similar to pheochromocytoma

  - Treatment = resection, can try neoadjuvant doxorubicin if unresectable

- o What is a nephroblastoma (Wilms tumor)?

  - Presentation: asymptomatic, hematuria, HTN, 10% are bilateral, average age 3 years old

    - Metastasizes to bone and lung (requires radiation)

  - Diagnosis = abdominal CT with replacement of renal parenchyma

    - WAGR = **W**ilms + **a**niridia + **G**U malformation + mental **r**etardation

  - Treatment = nephrectomy without rupturing (will upstage) + actinomycin and vincristine chemo

- o What are the features of a hepatoblastoma?

  - Elevated AFP

  - Treatment = resection, chemotherapy if unresectable

Hepatobiliary

- o Choledochal cyst **[See Hepatobiliary chapter]**

  - Thought to be caused by reflux of pancreatic enzymes in utero

  - 5 types- most common is Type I fusiform dilation of CBD

  - Treatment = resection, some require hepaticojejunostomy or liver TXP

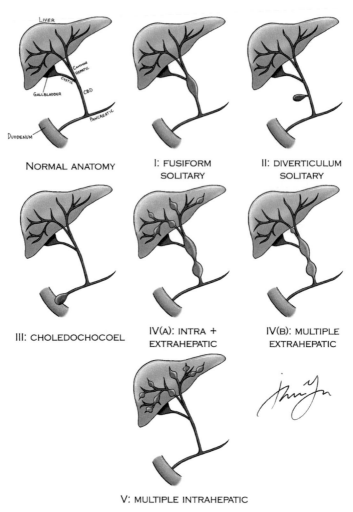

Figure 2 – Types of choledochal cysts

o What is biliary atresia?

- Most common indication for pediatric liver transplant

- Presentation: persistent neonatal jaundice

- Diagnosis = liver biopsy → periportal fibrosis, bile plug; US, cholangiography

- Treatment = Kasai (hepaticoportojejunostomy) is first step

if < 3 months of age → transplant

- 1/3 improve, 1/3 progress to transplant, 1/3 die

Thoracic

o What are the types of congenital lung disease?

- Pulmonary sequestration

  - Lung tissue that doesn't communicate with tracheobronchial tree with independent blood supply from aorta

  - Venous drainage can be systemic (extra-lobar) or pulmonary (intra-lobar)

  - Presentation: infection, abnormal CXR

  - Treatment = ligate arterial supply → lobectomy

- Congenital cystic adenoid malformation

  - Communicates with tracheobronchial tree (vs pulmonary sequestration)

  - Treatment = lobectomy

- Congenital lobar emphysema

  - Failure of cartilage development

  - Presentation: similar to tension PTX

  - Treatment = lobectomy

 Do not place a chest tube in congenital lobar emphysema.

- Bronchogenic cyst

  - Extrapulmonary cysts of bronchial tissue and cartilage

  - Presentation: mediastinal cystic mass

  - Treatment = resect

o What are the features of congenital diaphragmatic hernia?

- Two types:

- Bochdalek = most common, posterior

- Morgagni = rare, anterior

Bochdalek is back and to the left

- Most commonly left sided because the liver protects the right; usually both lungs are dysfunctional
- Associations: severe pulmonary HTN, cardiac and neural tube defects, malrotation
- Diagnosis = prenatal US, CXR will show bowel in chest
- Treatment = ventilation, inhaled nitric oxide, ECMO; stabilize → OR to run the bowel and repair defect

Neck

- ○ Where do branchial cleft cysts present?
  - Most commonly 2nd branchial cleft cysts which are on the middle of the anterior SCM
  - Treatment for all 3 branchial cleft cysts = resection
- ○ How do thyroglossal duct cysts present?
  - Midline (vs branchial cleft), goes through hyoid bone
  - Formed from abnormal descent of thyroid gland and may be patient's only thyroid tissue
  - Treatment = Sistrunk procedure → excision of cyst, tract, and hyoid bone to base of tongue
- ○ What is a cystic hygroma?
  - Lymphangioma, lymphatic malformation connecting to IJ
  - Presentation: Lateral neck in posterior triangle, soft, cystic, multi-loculated; gets infected
  - Treatment = resection

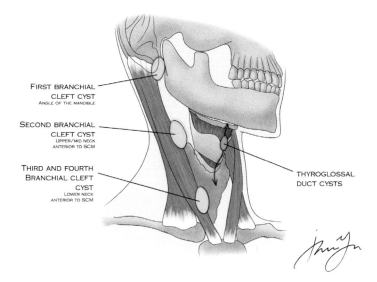

Figure 3 – Common cystic lesions of the neck

Quick Hits

- Which immunoglobulin crosses the placenta?
  - IgG

- Which immunoglobulin is transferred through breast milk?
  - IgA

- 1 month old with elevated AFP and beta-HCG. Diagnosis?
  - Sacrococcygeal teratoma - usually malignant after 2 months old

- Most common anterior mediastinal mass = teratoma
  - Most common overall mediastinal mass = neurogenic tumor (posterior mediastinum)

- 6-month-old with red lesions growing on face and scalp. Diagnosis and treatment?
  - Hemangioma will resolve by 8 years old, otherwise steroids or laser

- 13-year-old boy with large sunken area of chest?
  - Pectus excavatum → treat with strut if symptomatic
  - Pectus carinatum = pigeon chest, doesn't need correction (chest brace) unless emotional distress

20 BIOSTATISTICS

Descriptive Statistics

Mean	Average of data set. Can be skewed by extreme values. Mean of (1,6,2,6,7,4) is 4.33.
Median	Middle value of data set. Resistant to skew by extreme values. Median of (1,6,2,6,7,4) is 5 (in a dataset with even number of values, take the average of the two middle values).
Mode	Most common value of data set.
Range	Difference between the largest and the smallest value in the data set.

- Standard deviation describes how variable the points in the data set are compared to the mean of the data set.

- Normal distribution (aka Bell Curve or Gaussian distribution) – must be symmetric bell-shaped curve with the following standard deviations
  - 1 SD = 68% of samples are around the mean
  - 2 SD = 95% of samples are around the mean
  - 3 SD = 99.7% of samples are around the mean

- Other distributions:
  - Bimodal distribution: two peaks
  - Positively skewed distribution: peak is skewed toward the left, long tail on the right (mean > median > mode)
  - Negatively skewed distribution: peak is skewed toward the right, long tail on the left (mode > median > mean)

Statistical Testing

- Hypothesis testing
  - Null hypothesis (H_0) – there is no difference between two groups
  - Alternative hypothesis (H_1) – there is a difference between two groups

	Definition	Related concept
Type 1 error	H_0 is rejected when it is actually true. Thus H_1 is accepted when it is actually false. (False positive)	Alpha (α) is the probability of a type 1 error. This is the p-value, often set to 0.05 (5% chance of a type 1 error).
Type 2 error	H_0 is accepted when it is actually false. Thus H_1 is rejected when it is actually true. (False negative)	Beta (β) is the probability of a type 2 error. 1-β is the **power**, often set to 80%. Power increases with sample size.

- Common data structure scenarios and the appropriate tests:
  - Compare numerical means of two different groups: unpaired t-test (example: average BMI in sleeve versus bypass patients)
  - Compare two different numerical measurements taken from a single group of patients: paired t-test (example: BMI in patients before versus after getting a sleeve)
  - Compare numerical means of three or more groups: ANOVA (example: average BMI in sleeve versus bypass versus gastric band patients)
  - Compare categorical outcomes between two or more groups: chi-square test or Fischer's exact test (example: does VTE occur more often in patients who are obese?)

- o Identify and adjust for multiple potential factors contributing to a categorical outcome: multivariate logistic regression (example: in a large database, determine what variables contribute to incidence of infection)

- o Identify and adjust for multiple potential factors contributing to a numerical outcome: multivariate linear regression (example: in a large database, determine what variables contribute to total length of stay)

- o Identify difference in survivorship over time between two or more groups: Kaplan-Meier analysis (example: cancer survival in patients who received neoadjuvant versus adjuvant chemotherapy)

Types of Studies

- Case report – report of a single event or patient

- Case series – report of a small number of similar events or patients

- Prospective study – a research question and hypothesis is formed, then the data are collected

- Retrospective study – a research question and hypothesis are tested on existing data

- Observational study – analyze variables and outcomes in a non-controlled, natural group of subjects
  - o Cross-sectional study – analyze a population at a particular moment in time, to determine prevalence of factors and disease

  - o Cohort study – a population of subjects are analyzed to associate certain factors with an outcome; can be retrospective or prospective; can determine relative risk

  - o Case-control study – patients who had an outcome happen are compared to patients who did not have the outcome happen; these are always retrospective; cannot determine relative risk, only odds ratio

- Randomized controlled trial – rigorous study of an intervention done on two randomly assigned groups of subjects so that both groups are similar; these are always prospective
  - Single-blinded – the subjects do not know their group, but the researchers do
  - Double-blinded – neither the subjects nor the researchers know the groups

- Propensity-score-matched study – observational study that attempts to reduce confounding and be closer to a randomized controlled trial; cases are selected so that the subjects in both groups are similar across multiple factors

- Crossover study – each subject switches from one intervention to the other during the study, serving as their own control

- Systematic review – data from multiple studies are pooled
  - Meta-analysis – data from multiple studies are pooled with quantitative statistical methods

Clinical Drug Trials

- Preclinical – animal studies

- Phase 1 – small number of healthy subjects to test the pharmacology and side-effects of the drug

- Phase 2 – small number of diseased subjects to test the efficacy and dosing of the drug

- Phase 3 – randomized control trial to compare the drug to existing therapies

- Phase 4 – ongoing long-term trials after drug is approved to identify long-term side-effects and efficacy

Types of Risk

- Risk is the probability of a bad outcome

	Outcome did not happen	Outcome happened
Exposed to risk factor, or not treated with intervention	a	b
Not exposed to risk factor, or treated with intervention	c	d

Common risk-related concepts and how to calculate them

Absolute risk	Overall probability of the outcome	(a+b) / (a+b+c+d)
Relative risk	Probability of the outcome in exposed group compared to probability of outcome in non-exposed group	$\dfrac{(a/(a+b))}{(c/(c+d))}$
Odds ratio	Odds of the outcome in exposed group compared to odds of outcome in non-exposed group	$\dfrac{(a/b)}{(c/d)}$
Relative risk reduction	Proportion of decreased risk due to not being exposed	1 – relative risk
Absolute risk reduction	Difference in risk due to not being exposed	(c/c+d) – (a/(a+b))
Number needed to treat	Subjects that must be treated before one outcome is avoided	1 / absolute risk reduction

Diagnostic Testing

- Sensitivity – chance that a diseased person will test positive

- Specificity – chance that a non-diseased person will test negative
  - "SpIN and SnOUT" – Specific tests are good to **rule in**, Sensitive tests are good to **rule out**

- Positive predictive value – chance that a positive test result is correct

- Negative predictive value – chance that a negative test result is correct
  - Predictive values take into account the prevalence of the disease; sensitivity and specific do not

- Receiver-operating curve (ROC) – analyze what happens to sensitivity and specificity when you move the cut-off value of the test up or down
  - Larger area under the ROC curve means a better test

- How to calculate these:

	Diseased	Healthy	
Positive Test	True Positive (TP)	False Positive (FP)	$PPV = \dfrac{(TP)}{(TP) + (FP)}$
Negative Test	False Negative (FN)	True Negative (TN)	$NPV = \dfrac{(TN)}{(FN) + (TN)}$
	$Sensitivity = \dfrac{(TP)}{(TP) + (FN)}$	$Specificity = \dfrac{(TN)}{(FP) + (TN)}$	

Common Types of Bias

Lead-time bias	Falsely conclude that patients live longer when they were actually diagnosed earlier
Length-time bias	Falsely conclude that screening improves survival when actually screening only detects more benign disease courses
Surveillance bias	Falsely conclude that a disease is becoming more prevalent when actually we are testing for it more frequently
Recall bias	Subjects or researchers are more likely to remember certain factors than others (affects retrospective studies)
Allocation bias	A confounding factor affects the likelihood that a subject is assigned to a particular group in the study (solved by randomization)
Hawthorne effect	Subjects behave differently when they know they are being observed

Made in the USA
Monee, IL
17 June 2021

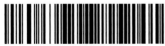